I knew that the moment I opened this book, I wouldn't be able to put it down. Aundi Kolber's words will meet you where you are, here in the present moment, shining light in the direction of connection and joy, in places where they are often a challenge to find. Her writing draws you into the depths as she gives you practical, grace-filled words of wisdom for every step. While reading this book, you will feel mirrored through Aundi's beautiful way of giving language to our experiences. You will be met in the wild of where you are while also receiving the tools you need so you can carry on for the rest of the journey.

MORGAN HARPER NICHOLS
Artist and poet

Try Softer is the book I've been searching for on the bookstore shelves. As someone who has been high-strung and "try-harder" since childhood, I've always wondered, *Why?* Why does my body feel on high alert even when my mind is quiet? Thankfully, Kolber's smart, informative approach and kind voice are here to help us all understand the complicated happenings between our heads, our hearts, and our bodies.

HAYLEY MORGAN
Author of *Preach to Yourself* and coauthor of *Wild and Free*

In a culture teeming with anxiety and feelings of being "not enough," Aundi is the friend and guide we need for this present moment. Packed with a perfect blend of relatable storytelling and practical methods, this book will be one

I return to and pass on to others. This is one of those rare lifelong reads you will pull out as a refresher course again and again.

HANNAH BRENCHER
Author of *Come Matter Here* and *If You Find This Letter*

Far too often the Christian recipe for abundant living involves mustering up more faith, doing more for God, and trying harder to make life work. In *Try Softer*, Aundi Kolber helps readers understand why such an approach never works and invites us to a radical new way of living— compassionately connected to ourselves, God, and others. With an extraordinary blend of personal vulnerability, scriptural acumen, and compelling neuroscience, Aundi ultimately shows readers that the abundant life we long for is less about striving and all about surrender.

MICHAEL JOHN CUSICK
CEO of Restoring the Soul and author of *Surfing for God*

In *Try Softer*, licensed therapist Aundi Kolber walks us toward the gentle understanding that our scars hold clues to our wholeness. Life is hard. Pain finds us. But as we learn to pay attention to our full selves, patiently excavating compassion from the rubble of critique, we will know healing. This kind, courageous book is right on time.

SHANNAN MARTIN
Author of *The Ministry of Ordinary Places* and *Falling Free*

ABOUT THE AUTHOR

AUNDI KOLBER is a licensed professional counselor (LPC), writer, and speaker living in Castle Rock, Colorado. She graduated from Denver Seminary in 2008 with an MA in community counseling. Aundi is the owner of Kolber Counseling, LLC, which was established in 2009. She has received additional training in her specialization of trauma- and body-centered therapies, including the highly researched and regarded eye movement desensitization and reprocessing (EMDR) therapy.

Aundi is passionate about the integration of faith and psychology, as well as its significance for the church today. She has written for *Relevant*, CT Women, (in)courage, the *Huffington Post*, Propel Sofia, Happy Sonship, and more. Aundi regularly speaks at local and national events, and she appears on podcasts such as *CXMH*, *The Upside Down Podcast*, *This Good Word with Steve Wiens*, and *Restoring the Soul*.

As a survivor of trauma and a lifelong learner, Aundi brings hard-won knowledge around the work of change, the power of redemption, and the beauty of experiencing God with us in our pain. She is happily married to her best friend, Brendan, and is the proud mom of Matia and Jude.

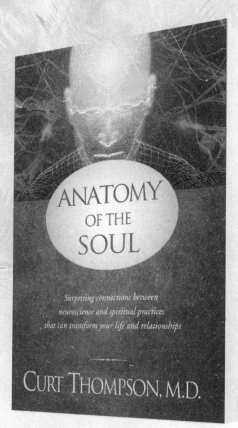

For those souls feeling alone in their suffering, *Try Softer* serves as a companion guide toward feeling connected and whole. Aundi Kolber's spiritual journey demonstrates that the way to transform pain is to surrender to the healing power of embodying compassion. *Try Softer* gives us faith and hope that light can be created out of darkness.

BARB MAIBERGER, MA, LPC
Founder of the Maiberger Institute, author of *EMDR Essentials: A Guide for Clients and Therapists*, and coauthor of *EMDR Therapy and Somatic Psychology: Interventions to Enhance Embodiment in Trauma Treatment*

Not since *The Body Keeps the Score* has a book made such a profound impact on my healing as a trauma survivor. *Try Softer* is a masterpiece, a seamless blend of competent clinical understanding and nurturing pastoral care. Aundi's unique dual perspective as both trauma therapist and trauma survivor gives her work an unparalleled depth of empathy, wisdom, and tenderness. She's created a powerful therapeutic tool that is an essential read not only for those who have been personally affected by trauma but also for therapists, pastors, educators, and caregivers.

STEPHANIE TAIT
Author of *The View from Rock Bottom*

Reading *Try Softer* feels a lot like exhaling. In a world that simultaneously pushes us to hustle and to hide our pain, Aundi Kolber wisely, tenderly, and skillfully offers us a new way forward. While it's certainly countercultural,

the message of *Try Softer* is both biblical and timely—
a presentation of the gospel that powerfully invites us to
live fully in the grace and healing Jesus freely offers.

ASHLEY ABRAMSON
Writer

For those exhausted from dragging their bodies through life
and white-knuckling their way through pain, Aundi Kolber
offers wise advice: Try softer. By learning to listen to your
body instead of fighting it, you can become more resilient
and more self-compassionate. *Try Softer* is exactly what a
stressed-out world needs to hear.

STEVE WIENS
Author of *Beginnings* and *Whole*

In a world that tells us we'd better be crushing it or killing
it if we want to make it, Aundi Kolber has a revolutionary
approach—trying softer. With grace, wisdom, and candor,
Try Softer gives us hope for a different way—lives of
connection and attention instead of competition and
distraction. If you're weary of trying so hard (who isn't?),
then try softer. You'll be glad you did.

NICOLE UNICE
Pastor, counselor, and author of *The Struggle Is Real*

TRY SOFTER

A Fresh Approach to Move Us out of

Anxiety, Stress, and Survival Mode—

and into a Life of Connection and Joy

AUNDI KOLBER MA LPC

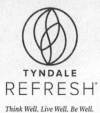

TYNDALE
REFRESH®

Think Well. Live Well. Be Well.

Visit Tyndale online at tyndale.com.

Visit Aundi at aundikolber.com.

Tyndale, Tyndale's quill logo, *Tyndale Refresh*, and the Tyndale Refresh logo are registered trademarks of Tyndale House Ministries. Tyndale Refresh is a nonfiction imprint of Tyndale House Publishers, Carol Stream, Illinois.

Try Softer: A Fresh Approach to Move Us out of Anxiety, Stress, and Survival Mode—and into a Life of Connection and Joy

Designed by Eva M. Winters

Published in association with Don Gates of the literary agency The Gates Group; www.the-gates-group.com.

For information about special discounts for bulk purchases, please contact Tyndale House Publishers at csresponse@tyndale.com, or call 1-855-277-9400.

The case examples in this book are fictional composites based on the author's professional interactions with dozens of clients over the years. All names are invented, and any resemblance between these fictional characters and real people is coincidental.

Library of Congress Cataloging-in-Publication Data

Names: Kolber, Andrea M., author.

Title: Try softer : a fresh approach to move us out of anxiety, stress, and survival mode-and into a life of connection and joy / Aundi Kolber.

Description: Carol Stream : Tyndale House Publishers, Inc., 2020. | Includes bibliographical references.

Identifiers: LCCN 2019034835 (print) | LCCN 2019034836 (ebook) | ISBN 9781496439659 (trade paperback) | ISBN 9781496439666 (kindle edition) | ISBN 9781496439673 (epub) | ISBN 9781496439680 (epub)

Subjects: LCSH: Stress management—Religious aspects--Christianity. | Stress (Psychology)—Religious aspects—Christianity. | Emotions—Religious aspects--Christianity. | Christianity—Psychology.

Classification: LCC BV4509.5 .K648 2020 (print) | LCC BV4509.5 (ebook) | DDC 248.4—dc23

LC record available at https://lccn.loc.gov/2019034835

LC ebook record available at https://lccn.loc.gov/2019034836

Printed in the United States of America

29	28	27	26	25	24	23
17	16	15	14	13	12	11

To Matia and Jude,
for lighting up my life with wonder and joy. May
you always know how deeply you are loved.

To Brendan,
for helping me find home again.

CONTENTS

LEARNING TO

TRY SOFTER IS NOT

A ONETIME EVENT

BUT A WAY

WE LEARN TO BE

WITH OURSELVES.

INTRODUCTION

I'D SEEN THE SIGNS MANY times before: Hunched shoulders. Clenched fists. Heavy sighs. Apologies for not being or doing enough. I'd come to notice these cues in others—I'm a therapist after all.

But this time I was the one in need of support. I was sitting in my counseling supervisor's office, feeling suffocated and exhausted, anxious and amped up. I thought the very fiber of my soul might give out if I tried to do or figure out one more thing.

It had been a tough week.

In reality, it had been a tough year. Most of my clients were adolescent girls or adult women, all of whom seemed to be experiencing an onslaught of heartbreak. Each day I listened to their accounts of abuse and pain, trying to help these women untangle their personal stories. At times I also calmed angry parents and soothed suicidal clients. The basic rule of being a therapist is that you should never work harder than your client, but I was breaking that rule ten times over and headed straight for burnout.

The truth was, I loved my job. I loved being able to come alongside my clients and guide them through the path of deep healing. But I was in a constant state of overwhelm. Having grown up in an intensely dysfunctional and chaotic family, I never fully learned how to hold the pain of others without internalizing it. My experience had taught me I wasn't allowed to. I didn't know how to listen to my own needs or the rhythms of my body. Consequently, when stressful and difficult weeks like this arose, I dealt with them the only way I knew how—by just trying to push through them, shaming myself in the process.

"John," I confessed to my supervisor, "I'm so worn out and tired. It just feels like no matter what I do, it's never enough. I feel like I'm failing my clients, like I'm not good enough to do this job."

John, whom I deeply respected, was already a seasoned therapist. He exuded wisdom and calm and regularly reminded me it was okay to be imperfect. As tears ran down my cheeks, John leaned forward in his chair for a moment and took a breath. Then, slowly, he rested his elbows on his knees and steepled his fingers, the way I often did with my own clients.

"Listen, Aundi," he said gently, "I'm curious about why you're so hard on yourself. You are providing the resources your clients need, and you are incredibly empathic. You're doing an excellent job." He cocked his head. "What would happen if you allowed yourself to release your grip on this situation?"

The empathy in John's voice felt soothing, and a part of me wanted to wholeheartedly embrace what he was saying. The other part of me was defensive; in fact, just considering his suggestion made my pulse race. *But how will anyone be okay if I don't care all the time?* my inner critic all but screamed. *If I'm not saving them, how will they survive?*

John leaned in again, sensing my ambivalence. "I'm not asking you to *stop* caring, Aundi . . . just to change *the way* you are caring. What I mean is . . . what if—just for a change—instead of trying harder, you tried . . . *softer?*"

I've got to be honest: At first blush, John's suggestion didn't sound like an awesome option—because what did it even mean? All I had ever learned was how to try harder. If I didn't push, everything would be terrible; everything would fall apart. The suggestion that there could be another way made my body feel tense with anger, a reflection of my twelve-year-old self—a girl riddled with the toxic stress of trying to keep everything together while her home life was constantly imploding. *Sure, John, "trying softer" sounds nice, but trying harder is how you survive.*

At the same time, I had to face the facts: Trying harder wasn't really working for me anymore. The strategies I had been using my entire life—hustling, overworking, overthinking, and constantly shifting to accommodate the dysfunction that surrounded me—they had kept me alive, yes, but now they were taking their toll. I felt less in control, not more; worse, not better; weary, not wise. The danger from my past was gone, but the patterns remained—and they were keeping me from being able to be truly present and pay attention to what matters most.

The day that I sat with John in his office totally changed the trajectory of my life because John was right: Pushing isn't always the answer.

Dear reader, there are truly times when the best, healthiest, most productive thing we can do is not to try *harder*, but rather to try *softer*: to compassionately listen to our needs so we can move through pain—and ultimately life—with more gentleness and resilience.

———

Perhaps you, too, know what it is like to feel overextended, overburdened, and overwrought, desperately clinging to the idea that if you just push hard enough, if you just try a little harder, you'll be able to regain control, soothe your anxious mind, and achieve some measure of success. And if you're anything like me, you may be feeling a little apprehensive: *Cool, Aundi, but I'm really busy. Who's going to do the hard stuff if I simply "try softer"? I don't wake up every morning wondering how I can sabotage my life by pushing so hard that there isn't any room for joy. It's just how it has to be.*

Friend, I hear you. But consider this: While hard work is valuable and necessary, there is a difference between pushing ourselves well and hurting ourselves by perpetuating harmful patterns.

We come by these tendencies honestly. We've learned to white-knuckle our way through life to armor up against pain and difficulty; we believe minimizing our wounds is the only way we'll be loved. We try to appear successful, productive, or simply okay on the outside, even when we're not okay on the inside. Our world overvalues productivity and others' opinions, so we learn to ignore the messages our bodies are giving us—through our emotions and physical sensations—and instead push through our pain and pretend we have it all together. Trying harder helps us feel safe in areas of our lives that may have felt overwhelming or out of control in the past.

What's more, we've been so socialized, parented, and wired to overfunction that we don't recognize when our bodies are stressed, traumatized, and exhausted until the consequences are dire. It's then, when anxiety and adrenaline have worn us down to a nub, that we may find ourselves depressed, exhausted, and disconnected.

You don't have to dismiss your pain here. You don't need to shrink it down or pretend living through it wasn't hard. You don't have to act like the shaming voices aren't still playing in your head, or like you're not still beating yourself up, or like the ways your needs were overlooked don't cut you daily. I'm not asking you to find the silver lining in your "hard." We know God is with us through it all, but that doesn't mean life hasn't cracked you open. It doesn't mean you haven't cried thousands of tears or spoken to yourself in ways you would never speak to another.

The wounds you have experienced are valid. Maybe no

one has ever said that to you, so I hope you'll receive this now: What's happened in your life matters.

I believe God's heart for us is outrageously gentle; and yet I believe He is calling us to more. While none of us are exempt from pain, we can learn to come out of survival mode and actually live. And isn't that what we all want—not to miss out on life? To have the tools, resources, and support we need to embrace the goodness? To see the people right in front of us? To live out Jesus' commandment to love our neighbor *as* ourselves (see Mark 12:31)? Imagine actually experiencing tenderness toward who you are—not just tolerating or enduring your life, your family, your relationships, your body, and your career, but truly finding ways to love and honor them.

This is what God created us for. This new way of being in the world is possible. Trying softer is the path that leads to true connection and joy. It begins when we mindfully listen to what's on the inside of us and let that influence how we look and act on the outside. It's an intentional shift toward paying compassionate attention to our own experiences and needs. Learning to try softer is not a onetime event but a way we learn to be with ourselves.

Like everything, trying softer isn't one-size-fits-all. We don't—and we shouldn't—approach it in exactly the same way either. For that reason, this book is meant not to be prescriptive but to offer you the tools and resources you can use to approach life with more self-compassion. This book is also not intended to diagnose mental health conditions or replace the valuable work of therapy. If you discover that it is bringing up unresolved trauma, anxiety, depression, or distress in other forms, I urge you to seek professional help.[1] My goal is that you learn to see yourself as your Creator sees you: as someone with infinite value who was created to be loved. And then I want you to live from that beautiful truth.

We'll start by looking back to see why you approach life the way you do; part 1 will take you through the process of understanding what circumstances hardwired you to white-knuckle your way through life. Drawing from the work of renowned scientists such as Daniel Siegel and Stephen Porges, you'll learn about the physiology of trying softer—why your body reacts to stress the way it does and how listening to your body can help you expand your ability to cope. Part 2 will introduce you to new practices and rhythms that will enable you to try softer in different areas of your life.

Dear reader, if you're anything like me and are all about finding solutions, you may be tempted to skip ahead to part 2. That's where the good, practical stuff is, right? That's the part that really matters.

With as much love as I can possibly send your way, I'm asking you not to do that. Here's why: Understanding why you came to live and behave the way you do is critical to implementing long-term change. If you approach the practices in part 2 as if they were a prescriptive fad, you aren't likely to stick with them. After all, you won't have the context to understand what deeper issues you need to address.

This work of trying softer isn't a quick fix to solve complex issues. Like the old adage says, "Give a man a fish, and you feed him for a day. Teach a man to fish, and you feed him for a lifetime."

My friend, I want to help you learn to fish. I want you to begin to develop a new awareness of your story and your wounds so you can attend to your pain with the same tenderness God does. If you're willing to do the work, learning to try softer will be a pathway to connecting with your truest, God-given self.

My hope is that the chapters ahead will be your invitation to embrace a more robust idea of what it means to be human—a person rooted in the wisdom and goodness of Jesus.

Will this work be vulnerable? It will.

Will it cost you something? Indeed, it will.

But I promise you that this sacred work will be worth it—because *you* are worth it; every single one of us is worth it. I want you to know what it's like to be fully alive—not because you'll be perfect or because it will be easy, but because this is what we were made for: a living, breathing, moving, feeling, connected, embodied life. This—all of this—is your birthright.

This is the "try softer" life.

PART 1

THE PROCESS OF BECOMING

THE PROCESS OF

BLOOMING IS

AS VALUABLE AS

THE FLOWER IT

PRODUCES.

CHAPTER 1

"BUT HOW LONG WILL IT TAKE?"

You either walk into your story and own your truth, or
you live outside of your story, hustling for your worthiness.
BRENÉ BROWN, *Rising Strong*

OLIVIA SAT ACROSS FROM ME in my counseling office and asked,
"But how long will it take to feel better?" Moments before,
she'd been sobbing, shoulders heaving, as she relayed the
deep pain she felt after being betrayed by a loved one. Her
breath had finally slowed, and she continued: "Isn't there
something I can do to get there quicker?"

Olivia and I had been working together for two months,
and while she reported feeling more hopeful overall and had
met a few small goals, she hadn't yet conquered what she felt
were her most significant issues.

Her question was one many of my clients have asked: *Isn't
there an easy fix to my problems? Is there any way we can just
wave a magic wand and be done?*

In a word, no.

I wish I could tell you yes; I really do. I want—for you and for me—to say that there's an easy fix, that all we have to do is follow three easy steps to truly heal. We don't like to sit in tension or process, especially when we know it may mean harder work. (I have yet to meet a person who is excited about the arc of change required to truly grow.) But in all I've learned as a therapist, and in all I've experienced as a human in this world—often the hard way—I believe the true work is slow and deep. That's how we'll truly heal.[1]

The work of trying softer begins when we release our desire for the quick fix and tend to the wounds underneath the surface. Otherwise, we're going to stay stuck. When losing weight doesn't make us feel valuable, when we discover that the people we've decided have all the answers are wrong, when anxiety returns minutes after we thought we'd handed our cares over to God—we may feel more hopeless than ever. This is why the ability to think about personal growth, people, issues, and relationships as a process matters a great deal. When people begin to understand that change happens in layers—and is rarely linear—it's as if someone took a grueling weight off them. They stand a bit straighter. Often they become a touch kinder to themselves and others. It's as if someone put a balm on their souls and gave them this message: "It takes as long as it takes. It's okay to be unfinished. It's absolutely normal to be imperfect. It doesn't mean you're doing anything wrong."

And what's more, God is neither surprised nor dismayed

at how slowly we progress. "We Christians, we have a saying about the Kingdom of God," writes Sarah Bessey. "It's now and it's not yet. We live in a tension. It's the tension of living our lives as Kingdom people, oriented around the life and teachings of our Jesus, a Christocentric people, in a world that is not yet redeemed. . . . It means that even though all things are made new, they are still in the process of *being made* new."[2]

The tension is where the real magic happens. As we accept the idea that process is part of what it means to be human, we are less intimidated by our unmet goals and are kinder to the wounded parts of ourselves.

Personal growth is a journey, not an event. It's a becoming. As author Brené Brown writes, "Owning our story and loving ourselves through that process is the bravest thing that we will ever do."[3]

Let's be brave together, friend.

THE POWER OF STORY

Unfortunately, many of us have been taught—either consciously or unconsciously—that our stories and our experiences don't matter. Perhaps if we simply "buck up," our problems will magically resolve. Or possibly we just need to forget what happened and "let it go."

That is the approach Erica, a mother of two and part-time account manager in a marketing firm, tried to take. She is smart, capable, and kind. She appears to have it all together, so people are always asking for her help. In turn, she attempts to offer more than she has to give. Growing up, Erica learned that she didn't have much of a choice. The message she received from demanding parents was that no matter how bad she felt on the inside, it was essential to uphold the image of a successful family. This cemented her belief that she had to appear okay even if she wasn't. Throughout her childhood and adolescence, Erica constantly battled shame, feeling that she was just too sensitive and too much because she couldn't keep her emotions from bubbling up.

Now as an adult, Erica finds herself constantly ignoring signs of hunger, stress, sadness, or the terrible pain in her neck and back—pushing down discomfort because she's promised herself she won't be too much anymore. At the office, she's productive, but she feels as if she is always one moment away from breaking. What if she forgets to reply to that important email? What if her work doesn't meet expectations? What if . . . ?

Erica runs on constant anxiety and adrenaline at work, and when she comes home, she is fried and emotionally overwhelmed. She is often trying new techniques to help her better manage her life, but they never stick. When she takes a rare moment to reflect at the end of the day, she recognizes that she's her own worst critic—which probably isn't healthy—but who has the time or energy to be kind to themselves?

Like the ever-elusive quick fix, ignoring, pretending, or numbing something doesn't usually resolve our pain. Instead, we must find ways to validate that our stories are real and—although we may not like parts of them—that they are ours.

Such an approach is diametrically opposed to what we've been taught. Instead of trying so hard to forget, we try softer by becoming engaged, attentive observers of our bodies, minds, and spirits so that we can give each of those parts what it actually needs to heal. From a psychological and physiological perspective, the more disconnected we are from our lived experience, the more overwhelmed or numb to our lives we'll be. Research has shown us, in fact, that having cohesive stories matters for our emotional wellness.[4]

As a trauma-informed therapist, I don't consider stories to simply be abstract concepts or ethereal ideas, but instead the neurobiological framework through which we experience life—for better or worse. Simply put, stories—or the compilation of events, emotions, sensations, ideas, and relationships we've experienced—are held in our minds and bodies, and they affect how we see our world. The templates some of us live from confirm that we are relatively safe and loved, and though we are imperfect, we are still capable. Others among us have been hardwired through our experiences to believe that we are not enough or that we're shameful, unlovable, or any number of other untruths.

The stories we weave and the meaning we make from them create templates for how we understand God, life, others, and ourselves. Regardless of the frameworks we carry, choosing to care for and nurture the whole history of who we are is connected to the way we were made to thrive.

What does it look like if we're disconnected from our stories—and why would we want to disconnect in the first place? Typically, it's because some parts of them feel disturbing, or at least uncomfortable. As a result, we may want to minimize or numb the pain we've been through, the significance of our wounds, or the intensity of our discomfort. In my own life, I often attempt to distance myself from pain in the way I speak about it, apologizing to people for my feelings or for being a "burden." It's only when I acknowledge that my experience is valid that I have the ability to do something with my discomfort.

When we deny the reality of our experiences, we don't become more of who God designed us to be, but less. There's no way to have cohesive stories unless we truly embrace all of it: the good, the hard, the bittersweet, the sad, the joyful, the lonely, and the painful. It all counts.

If we know something else to be true, it's this: God is a curator and keeper of stories. Psalm 56:8 says, "You keep track of all my sorrows. You have collected all my tears in your bottle. You have recorded each one in your book" (NLT). God is invested in the entire arc of our humanity. He made us this way, and it's no accident that our physiology connects with his design. Learning how to be "with" our stories—in our bodies, without becoming overwhelmed by or numbing our past experiences—is the way we will learn how to actually handle and move through the grief and anxiety that come up. It's also the way we will learn to write new endings that are true to ourselves.

I've watched this transformation take place in many people's lives as they've become compassionate witnesses to the pain they've experienced or the parts of themselves that have felt too much. As they came to terms with their life stories, each person learned to try softer in a slightly different way:

- Gretchen began to acknowledge the grief she felt over parents who were critical and inconsistent in her childhood. Instead of shaming herself over wounds that still hurt, she learned to speak kindly to herself when she felt stuck.

- Pete began paying mindful attention to the tension he felt even when he was away from the office, which kept him from engaging with his family when he was home. By setting boundaries around his work and email life, he was able to be truly present with his family.

- Gina learned to pay compassionate attention to herself so she could recognize when she was pushing herself far beyond her capacity in an effort to make other people happy. Now she's learning how to be okay with other people's disappointment. She also spends more time with people who honor her limits.

- For Tim, trying softer meant getting curious about his disconnection from just about every emotion—except anger—and then letting himself see what might be behind this shutdown of most of his feelings.

- Monique began taking time to notice her body's cues around pain and hunger. No longer does she try to push through the whole day starving and tired, but instead she paces her life differently so she can feed and care for herself. She also takes short breaks simply to notice what she actually feels.

- Elaina learned to reach out to friends and family when she felt exhausted and alone rather than trying to act as if she were always okay.

Although trying softer looks a bit different for each of them, they are all listening to themselves in new ways. In fact, paying compassionate attention to themselves is what tells them how to move forward.

SLOW DOWN

Reader, it's incredibly normal to want to be finished with growth and healing. I get it. I remember when I first started meeting with a counselor back when I was in graduate school. Bless my heart, I went in ready to white-knuckle my way through all the pain. "Let's just get it over with" was my mantra. I figured there had to be a quick way to achieve the perceived perfection that would finally help me feel calm and at peace. In a sense, this desire to rush the process was the opposite of honoring my story. I wanted to hurry past it because it was extremely painful in parts. The reality is, it has taken years of trauma therapy to be fully present with elements of my life that caused deep wounds. I tell you this because my experience is actually quite normal. None of us are exempt—but some cuts may be deeper than others.

So what does owning all of your story look like? For Erica, learning to tell her story means she has to honestly acknowledge where she is avoiding or minimizing pain. It also means that when something feels too overwhelming for her to consider in a particular moment, she or her therapist takes a break from exploring that part further until she feels ready to address it more fully. Over time, Erica can develop the ability to embrace all parts of her story.

Just as there's no way to rush a flower to bloom, we cannot go beyond the stage we are in—we have to move at the pace that feels doable to us. This is why I invite you to respect the intensity of your experience and to remember that the in-between is sacred too. If I've learned anything, it may be that the *way* we do something matters as much as *what* we do. The process of blooming is as valuable as the flower it produces.

If you're like me or Erica, parts of your story may bring up pain—there's no shame in that. It's simply a sign that it may be good to pause or slow your pace when you delve into difficult pieces. Sometimes I tell my clients, "Let's dance

White-Knuckling 101

We "white-knuckle" when we consciously or unconsciously ignore internal warning signs from our minds and bodies to cope with situations that are overwhelming or disturbing. Often we learn to overfunction not out of choice but as a way to survive. This approach then carries over into everyday life because we don't know a different way.

We white-knuckle when we . . .

· ignore signs of pain, hunger, or exhaustion;
· minimize our emotions (*Oh, it's not that bad*);
· find ourselves overwhelmed by big emotions that we've ignored too long;
· numb our emotions (Netflix binge, anyone?);
· say yes when we mean no;
· bounce between feeling motivated by and then overwhelmed by adrenaline; or
· go through seasons of profound exhaustion, depression, or numbness because we've been overfunctioning.

with your story." I mean that they may step into their stories and find them tolerable for a moment, but if they notice themselves becoming overwhelmed, it's absolutely appropriate to take a metaphorical or physical step back. That's process. How might you do this? First, give yourself permission to fully shift out of your story for a bit. For example, pop a mint in your mouth and notice the flavors or the tingling on your tongue. Turn on your favorite song and sing along at the top of your lungs. Or arrange to meet a friend or two for coffee and let yourself receive their warmth.

The truth is that for many of us, embracing our stories is the work of a lifetime. This idea of honoring our lived history is more about an internal posture that keeps us open and curious to the nuances than it is about completing a task.

The great thing is, you don't have to be done embracing your story to come along with me on this journey of trying softer. If I were sitting across from you, I would tell you, "I do not want you to white-knuckle through your story; that's not what we're here for. Instead, think of our work in a circular way: We'll begin here, we'll move forward, and sometimes we'll come back to a place of examining our stories—not because we'll be stuck, but because this is all part of the process of healing."

The goal of trying softer isn't to bring about a quick fix, but to empower us with the freedom to live in the here and now while still honoring and tending to the wounds of our stories that have kept us disconnected from our experiences.

TRY SOFTER

As we prepare to embark on this journey, I invite you to consider a few questions that will give you a starting point for embracing your story. Remember that some parts may feel especially difficult to spend time with; for now, feel free to simply note them.

1. On a piece of paper, create a timeline of your life. Write down the major events first and then the more ordinary ones. What events stand out to you most? Spend as much or as little time on this exercise as you feel comfortable with. You may decide to use different colors to highlight different types of events, such as pink for transitions, green for losses, blue for accomplishments, red for experiences that felt overwhelming, etc.

2. Spend time considering your story as you feel able. In what ways have you tried to minimize or divorce yourself from your story? Are there any events you don't feel you have the ability to spend much time with? Are there any areas you are tempted to minimize that leave you with a visceral feeling of yuck? Perhaps mark these with an asterisk or write a note beside them on your timeline.

3. Where in your story do you desire to see change or healing but feel unable to move forward?

4. Where in your story do you feel proud of yourself for what you've made it through or how you've adapted to change?

5. When you feel ready, show your timeline to someone with whom you feel emotionally safe (friend, spouse, therapist, pastor, etc.).

WHEN WE CAN LOVINGLY
TURN TOWARD OUR PAIN,
EXPRESSED IN VARIOUS
WAYS BY OUR BODIES,
WE OFTEN BEGIN TO FIND
WE HAVE CHOICES WE
COULDN'T SEE BEFORE.

CHAPTER 2

MIND YOUR BRAIN

Our bodies are prophets.
They know when things are out of whack and they say so.
BARBARA BROWN TAYLOR, *An Altar in the World*

VERONICA, WHO STRUGGLED with both anxiety and severe disconnection, was distressed because she felt unable to accept the love she knew her husband wanted to offer her. She often bristled at his simplest requests.

"I don't understand it," she told me. "One minute Jason is asking me if I can pick up something from the store, and the next minute I'm feeling totally foggy—or even worse, I'm hyperventilating. I have this awful sense of dread, and it's as if I'm watching myself and not connected to my body. I want to feel closer to my husband, but I'm just so scared."

She told me that she felt both stressed out and disconnected from just about everything in her life—including her husband—and that she shut down whenever any difficult conversation began. Later I learned that, as a child, Veronica never knew how her father, a war veteran with post-traumatic stress disorder (PTSD), would behave when he returned home from work. In fact, his moods were so wildly unpredictable that everyone would cower until they knew what frame of mind he was in. On good nights, he would ask to see Veronica's homework and offer her praise and the smile she loved. These were the nights Veronica lived for—and she would tread carefully and watch what she said, hoping to please him and not mess anything up.

Usually once or twice a week, however, something small—like a broken dish—would set her father off, and he would yell for hours, exploding with cutting insults and ferocious anger. On some occasions the police were called because he had thrown the family's clothes into the street and yelled at the neighbors. Veronica's mother, a survivor of childhood trauma, would retreat into a depression for days afterward, forcing the kids to fend for themselves. At other times, Veronica's mother was loving and available—but in the terrifying moments when Veronica needed her most, she wasn't there.

Several years later, Veronica's father received treatment for his PTSD, and the intensity and fear in their home lessened. However, the family never spoke about what had happened since they didn't want anyone to think less of them—especially at church—so Veronica always felt she had to keep it a secret. By the time Veronica experienced sexual violence in high school, she had already internalized the belief that these types of issues were not to be discussed and that her feelings didn't matter. As a result, she didn't report the event or seek any support afterward.

During our sessions, Veronica was able to tell me the specifics of many events from her childhood, but she had only faint memories of the nights when her dad's anger was bad, as well as the event during high school. A terrible stomachache would suddenly appear whenever we delved into those topics.

Because Veronica had adapted to previous frightening experiences by alternately white-knuckling through them and dissociating from them,[1] those responses became her default whenever hard things came up—even after she'd grown up and left home.

OUR BODIES: THE GREAT COMMUNICATORS

Each of our lives tells a story, and our bodies were created to give us valuable information as we experience those stories. That is why whenever I work with clients in therapy, one of the key elements I'm always tracking is their autonomic nervous systems (ANS),[2] which is essentially the part of the nervous system that controls unconscious functions like breathing, heart rate, and visceral responses to threat. It's also important to me to empower my clients, like Veronica, with this knowledge. When we can lovingly turn toward our pain, expressed in various ways by our bodies, we often begin to find we have choices we couldn't see before.

The ANS has two parts—the sympathetic and the *para*-sympathetic. The sympathetic is what drives our fight/flight response by stimulating cortisol and adrenaline to mobilize us to fight or flee danger.[3] Additionally, a lesser-known but equally significant reaction from the sympathetic nervous system is the fawn response. In this state, our bodies attempt to neutralize prolonged danger by pleasing or accommodating others rather than acknowledging our discomfort.[4] This explains why Veronica would do everything possible to keep her dad and others happy so they wouldn't blow up or be displeased, which she had learned could lead to danger.

It's important to understand that in fight/flight/fawn, our bodies respond with corresponding levels of arousal to perceived threats. In some instances we may feel only mildly activated, whereas in other situations we may be hyper-vigilant and feel totally out of control. When this happens, the higher-thinking parts of our brains become so disconnected from our actions that two things can occur. First, our bodies unconsciously respond to the threats in the best ways they can—without necessarily consulting the higher brain. Second, we may behave completely contrary to our "normal" selves in order to deal with real or perceived dangers.

Conversely, the *para*sympathetic nervous system—which is often referred to as "rest and digest"—is in play when we are in a relaxed state. However, another function of the parasympathetic nervous system is to shift the body into a "freeze" state as a way of coping with terror when a person perceives they are in danger and there is no escape. This is our bodies' way of trying to protect us from actual or perceived impending doom without consulting our thinking brains. When the freeze response is activated, it occurs on a continuum from mild fogginess or not feeling present to fainting or physical collapse.

Many of us who've relied on white-knuckling as a way of getting through life don't realize that in addition to feeling anxious and overwhelmed, we may be dealing with elements of dissociation. For years, I thought I simply struggled with anxiety. It wasn't until I began to observe and experience my body differently that I began to see that at times I also experienced dissociation, another name for the "freeze" response.

When I was in college, I remember returning to my dorm after a terribly chaotic weekend with my family. My parents had fought and threatened each other, and I spent the two days on continual high alert. I felt shame and the constant, familiar sense that the bottom of my life could fall out, and no one would be there to catch me. When I arrived back at my small dorm room, I wondered if the grief might swallow me. It seemed that no one could understand how alone I felt. It was like a heavy blanket had descended on me. I assumed it was depression, but I now understand it was dissociation. In essence, my parasympathetic nervous system was trying to help me detach from the parts of my life that were overwhelming. I longed to sleep or zone out because the world felt like far too much, and I simply didn't have what it took to face it.

When we learn the way our environments and relationships shape the stories we hold in our bodies—and that we can find more nurturing, effective ways to care for ourselves as we move through difficulties—it becomes easier to be gentle with pain when it shows up.

EMPOWERED TO UNDERSTAND OURSELVES

A significant part of learning to try softer comes from recognizing that old wounds may be causing us to live in fight/flight/fawn or freeze even once we're safe. For this reason, although our brains are complex, even a base-level understanding of how they function is empowering. Learning about the choices we have for *how to respond* to our own bodies before they're in full-blown crisis can help us to make choices that better reflect our true selves. If we've experienced a history of distress, shame, or overwhelm, we may feel that the sensations in our bodies and thoughts in our minds are simply happening to us instead of having a sense of control over how we respond to our lives and wounds.

When I understand why my brain is reacting the way it is, I become empowered to validate the underlying need and then work on changing the situation. With that said, let's consider the main parts of our "triune brains,"[5] starting with the base and moving to the top.

Brain Stem

ASKS THE CORE QUESTION, *AM I SAFE?*

The most primitive part of your brain, the brain stem, works with your limbic system to manage functions like sleep, sex drive, breathing, and arousal. It also determines how your body will respond to threats (fight/flight/fawn or freeze). When you're reacting to what your brain stem is telling you, you may (or may not) notice urges to do something, but you may not know why you have those impulses. For example, you might walk into a room painted a certain color and suddenly want to leave without any conscious reason. Upon further work in therapy, you may recall that you were constantly verbally abused in a room that precise shade of green—and realize that your body, indeed, remembers.[6] Ignoring your body can result in rigid and compulsive behavior because the brain stem is acting from a place of survival without the support of your thinking brain to help regulate it.

Prefrontal Cortex
(facilitates higher-level thinking)

Can I learn? Can I problem-solve? Can I regulate? Can I empathize?

Limbic System
(assigns meaning to emotions; coordinates with brain stem to assess danger)

Am I loved? Is this good or bad?

Brain Stem
(connects brain to information provided by body)

Am I safe?

Limbic System

ASKS THE CORE QUESTIONS, *AM I LOVED? IS THIS GOOD OR BAD?*

The limbic system[7] is more advanced than the brain stem. Its main roles include experiencing attachment with others (via the entire system), creating certain types of memories (via the hippocampus and amygdala), and working with the brain stem to regulate hormones that contribute to a response to physical and emotional threats (via the hypothalamus and pituitary gland). Additionally, the amygdala plays an important role in the fear response. For example, if you were about to be hit by a car, your amygdala—without a conscious thought—would likely assess the situation and alert the systems of your body to get out of the way. Finally, the entire limbic system is where your emotions, and the meanings you make from them, live. Based on prior experiences, this part of your brain determines what type of emotion is evoked in you.

Cortex and Prefrontal Cortex

ASKS THE CORE QUESTIONS, *CAN I LEARN? CAN I PROBLEM-SOLVE? CAN I REGULATE? CAN I EMPATHIZE?*

Lobes within your cortex influence your physical perception and motor functions. This part of your brain even allows you "to think about thinking."[8] The most advanced part of your brain—called the prefrontal cortex (PFC)—continues developing into early adulthood. The PFC is what enables you to be aware of and then process your emotions and experiences. Though nestled within your cortex, it is positioned only a synapse away from the brain stem and limbic system.[9] Practically this means it can bring into awareness what is going on in those parts of your brain, including the sensory information the brain stem receives from the rest of the body.

In order for you to try softer, you must be aware of what is going on in your body, and the PFC allows you to do just that.

Your brain develops from the bottom up[10] because your body prioritizes baseline functions like breathing, heart rate, and a sense of safety (brain stem). The brain then begins developing the need to attach to a caregiver (limbic system). It forms its unconscious functions and attachment circuitry before it forms the ability to experience empathy, think with nuance, and problem-solve (cortex).

However, when your body goes into fight/flight/fawn or freeze, blood flow is directed away from the PFC so that the energy can be distributed elsewhere. When you live only from the brain stem, everything else is "offline." This adaptive reflex is incredibly helpful when you are about to be hit by a car or need to escape a burning building, but it can be problematic if you're trying to make dinner plans with a friend. Your brain wants to be sure the person in front of you is safe before it is able to concentrate on social planning.

When the PFC is online, information from all three parts of your brain is linked, which is known as *vertical integration*. You can then pay attention and respond to the information your whole brain is giving you, which is essential to trying softer.

When I was overwhelmed by the dysfunction of my family, I had no framework for how my brain worked, so when the lower parts of my brain gave me tons of information, like a racing heart, shortened breath, a sense of dread, and the desire to numb myself, I had no way to understand those signals. Without a proper lens, I thought I was just weak, sinful, or bad. I didn't understand that I had gone into a state psychologists call *hyper*arousal (most commonly associated with fight and flight).

But now as an adult, trying softer has helped me recognize that during my childhood, my limbic system was highly triggered by feeling alone and unsafe. I have learned through counseling to stay connected to my whole brain while also paying attention to the parts that still hurt. In doing this, I can notice when I have a sense of dread, and rather than ignoring, stifling, or shaming myself, I can become compassionate and curious instead.

Similarly, when Veronica told me she'd lost touch with time whenever things had become scary around her dad and when she'd experienced sexual violence, I helped her understand that the top of her brain, which would have allowed her to remain present to herself and her body, had not been available to her. Rather than sending her into hyperarousal, as my childhood trauma had done to me, she went into a state known as *hypo*arousal (typically associated with freeze/dissociation). She had been truly terrified back then, but now that she was an adult, her body was still wired to rely on the same coping techniques whenever an event or person triggered a fearful response in her. Once again, she froze.

When we're anxious, we may have similar responses. Although we may feel that we are solving problems by thinking about them, if we are in fight-or-flight mode, we are not able to connect to the systems of our bodies that allow us to truly problem-solve. We get stuck ruminating on our problems instead.

BIG T OR LITTLE T: TRAUMA IS TRAUMA

Stories like Veronica's and mine are not uncommon. Many of us, at some point or another, have had experiences that felt so overwhelming or threatening to our nervous systems that

When I'm in HYPERAROUSAL (fight/flight/fawn), I may feel:	When I'm in HYPOAROUSAL (freeze), I may feel:
• overwhelmed with adrenaline;	• sluggish;
• my heart racing;	• depressed;
• physical shaking/trembling;	• suddenly exhausted;
• the urge to move my body—either away from or toward the stressful event;	• foggy/zoned out;
• angry;	• paralyzed—frozen to the spot;
• out of control;	• numb/shut down;
• scared;	• disconnected from the world; or
• anxious; or	• as though I'm watching myself.
• the need to overaccommodate or to please people.	

our brains encoded that information on a spectrum from disturbing to outright traumatic. Although many people assume that only literal war stories result in trauma, I work from a broader definition.

After all, whether our bodies experience something as disturbing or traumatic is based as much on our perception of that event as on the event itself.[11] For instance, two people may be involved in a car accident. One may get through it with few lingering effects, while the other experiences flashbacks and hypervigilance whenever she gets back in her car. What matters most is how a person *experiences* a situation.[12]

A traumatic event includes anything that overwhelms a person's nervous system and ability to cope.[13] When this happens, the body is unable to metabolize[14] the stress or event, and the disturbing experience becomes "stuck" in the person's nervous system.

These overwhelming experiences of stress can turn into big T trauma, which leads to post-traumatic stress disorder. Certain experiences, such as sexual violence and serious injury, or witnessing someone undergo sexual assault, a life-threatening injury, or death, are such distinct personal violations that they are always classified as big T trauma.[15] Little t trauma, on the other hand, results from events that would not normally be considered catastrophic, but that can still overwhelm or seriously challenge a person's ability to cope and lead to symptoms similar to PTSD.[16]

One hallmark of both big T and little t trauma is that the memory of the event isn't normal. Instead of recalling something as though it had happened in the past—as if we were looking at a photograph while thinking about it—we experience it as though it were happening in the present. Depending on the specifics of the trauma, we may experience a spectrum of associated sights, smells, emotions, beliefs, and sensations when it is triggered. For example, a little t trauma connected to feeling shamed in childhood will likely bring up a visceral experience of feeling significantly younger and worthless, but not necessarily specific smells and pictures.

On the other hand, a war veteran with PTSD may experience a flashback that includes much more sensory information.[17] In either type of situation, the experience isn't integrated with the prefrontal cortex like a normal memory; therefore, we don't have a link to the coping skills, calming memories, or healthy connections that could help us navigate the situation in present time.

You may have noticed that big T trauma and little t trauma feel eerily similar. This is because they are on the same spectrum. This does not minimize in any way the pain of a big T traumatic event that leads to PTSD. But little t trauma carries its own weight. Leading neuroscientist and researcher Stephen Porges says we should "ask not about the event, but focus on the individual reaction or response. . . . The point that we have to understand is that when a person has a reaction or response to trauma, the body interprets the traumatic event as a life threat."[18]

Part of the reason I white-knuckled my way through life for so many years is because that was the way my body dealt with chronic, unprocessed little t emotional trauma. It was a valid response to an overwhelming and unstable home. For years I didn't believe my experiences were "bad enough" to count, so I didn't see myself as a survivor of trauma, even though I had the same symptoms. It wasn't until I learned about the nervous system and gained additional training that I understood how significant it is to experience trauma in childhood—and how it can affect us long after.

So while not everyone is walking around with PTSD, almost everyone has experienced little t traumas.[19] For

Big T Trauma	I may experience or feel:	Little t Trauma
Witnessing or experiencing any of the following events can result in post-traumatic stress disorder:* · a life-threatening situation · sexual violence · serious injury · natural disaster	· triggered by anything that reminds me of the event; · emotional or visual flashbacks that bring up the same emotions or sensations as during the event; · a desire to avoid thoughts or feelings related to the event; · nervous system dysregulation (anxiety/depression/anger/fear related to the event); or · a change in core belief about myself related to the event (e.g., I'm bad; It's my fault).	Little t trauma includes any experience that overwhelms your ability to cope and continues to feel disturbing—situations such as · being the target of bullying; · having absent/estranged parents; · being the target of verbal/emotional abuse; · going through a bad breakup; · experiencing racism or discrimination; · experiencing grief or loss; · experiencing intense transitions; · growing up in poverty; or · undergoing medical procedures.

*Please keep in mind that this is not meant as the full diagnostic criteria for PTSD. If you suspect you may have PTSD, please see a mental health professional for a full evaluation.

example, very capable people who grew up with hypercritical parents may find themselves constantly second-guessing themselves, lacking boundaries, and overworking. The man who experienced incessant bullying may find himself always needing to be tough, even when those closest to him long to see his tender side. The woman who grew up with a mother entrenched in addiction may find herself crushed by the death of a beloved pet that was her closest connection. Or the new mom who felt alone and neglected as a child may struggle to bond with her newborn.

Consider how Veronica's experience of chronic little t trauma in her childhood prevented her from reaching out for support when she encountered sexual violence. Without the resources needed to process such a terrifying event, that incident was made even more traumatic. This is the nature of trauma: It doesn't simply go away but instead informs how we exist in the world whether we acknowledge it or not.

Remember Erica from chapter 1, who also white-knuckled her way through much of life? Most people wouldn't think of Erica as a survivor of trauma. But having caregivers who chronically shame or suppress your emotional experiences results in a type of emotional trauma. No wonder, then, that as an adult she was plagued by a primal anxiety and disconnection that she couldn't seem to correct.

One way we might think about the difference between big T trauma and little t trauma is to compare a person with a deep knife wound who needs immediate emergency room care with someone who gets a paper cut at the office. One paper cut might hurt and even cause some difficulties in daily life, but it's not necessarily going to stop that person from living. However, a person who suffers a thousand paper cuts but is told those injuries are nothing is unlikely to ever stop to care for them. She may even assume that she is weak or lacks character as her pain mounts. At some point, however, her hand is likely to become infected, and she, too, will need to head to the emergency room. Whether the trauma is big or little, people find great relief when they receive validation that their wounds need care.

Do you see how this work can get complex?

When left unaddressed and without proper support and resources, these little t traumas can significantly affect our nervous systems. This is especially true if those events occurred from birth to age eighteen, when the brain is particularly malleable. Research confirms that adverse childhood experiences, especially in the absence of a loving and consistent caregiver to help alleviate the stress, or in the presence of a caregiver who caused the stress, can negatively shape a person's emotional, physical, and spiritual health. Studies show that the more of these events children experience, the higher the likelihood they will suffer from chronic illness, chronic pain, mental health issues, addiction, and relational issues.[20]

REFRAME

For those of us who've felt out of control, disconnected from our bodies and emotions, or unable to live out what we know to be true, survival may sometimes be our only goal. Yet as heavy a topic as trauma is, I'd like to offer you a reframe: Whenever hard things activate us, our bodies are showing us they want to move toward healing and integration. As difficult as triggers can be, with the proper support and resources, we can learn to integrate those experiences into who we are in a healthy way; in essence, this is the work of owning our stories. Often this requires the support of a therapist coming alongside us, but the try-softer approach I introduce in this book can provide a framework for how to move into growth in a gentle way.

To put it concisely, we integrate our minds by making sure we have adequate resources to reprocess the painful material into a memory as we would a normal event.[21] Just because we've gone through something overwhelming doesn't mean we must stay stuck there; difficult experiences don't have to become trauma. However, we must learn to listen to the information our bodies are telling us so we can process the painful events.

In my own life, for example, I've had to become aware of my tendency to want to overaccommodate whenever someone has expectations of me. I now know this is because when I was a child, expectations were fraught with pain and shame. Yet the process of trying softer has taught me to notice when my body becomes activated to what feels like a potential threat. As I pay compassionate attention to my whole self, I can better determine if this feeling is warranted or if instead I need to help regulate my body and remind myself that I have choices now that I never had before; I can set limits and use my voice in any way I need. I remind myself that my fear is valid but that I do not need to allow it to drive me anymore. I am safe now.

This sacred invitation to honor our pain is holy work and a journey to which we are all called. To appreciate how our physiology is designed to adapt in threatening situations, I often view it from the perspective that we have a Creator who gives us what we need to make it through, to live another day. As the book of James tells us, "Every good and perfect gift is from above" (1:17, NIV). I believe that the desire of our bodies to survive is a gift.

And yet these unconscious responses to threat (fight/ flight/fawn or freeze) are meant only to be temporary. They are meant to get us through danger. They are meant to protect our souls and essence. Let's be absolutely clear: There is no shame in surviving. But merely surviving is a far cry from living fully alive, and that, dear reader, is our ultimate goal with trying softer.

TRY SOFTER

It can be both empowering and overwhelming to recognize how trauma may be influencing your life. In this exercise you will strengthen your tolerance for difficult parts of your story by building your positive resources first and connecting to them in a visceral way.

1. Look back at your timeline from the exercises in the previous chapter. Pick an event or experience that you feel proud of or that reminds you of your true self. Another option is to recall someone or something that has felt supportive to you (e.g., a teacher, a particular place, even a good book).

2. Take a moment to visualize your body in your mind's eye. Now, as though a laser were scanning your body for information, notice where you are experiencing any sensations, tingling, feelings of calm, or pleasant emotions. As you notice these, take a moment and simply place a hand on those parts of your body. Notice if any words or phrases pop up in your mind as you do this, such as "I'm capable" or "I'm strong." If you feel comfortable doing so, perhaps say to your body, "Thank you for giving me information. I am listening now." If this continues to feel pleasant, stay with this practice for thirty seconds to a minute, remembering you can stop whenever you want.

AGAIN & AGAIN

HE COMES FOR US;

HE LOVINGLY FINDS US.

HE MAKES A WAY

WHERE THERE

WAS NO WAY.

CHAPTER 3

ATTACHED:
WHY OUR EARLIEST RELATIONSHIPS MATTER

---

i carry your heart with me
(i carry it in my heart)
E. E. CUMMINGS

AS YOU MOVE toward a more authentic, gentler way to be in the world, I think it's important you know some of my story.

What's my stake in the game?

Why do I care so much about this process?

Like most people's stories, mine starts long ago, and it has much pain and trauma and many threads of beauty woven in deep. And if I'm honest, my story begins before I do, with the story of my mother. I want to share the context of her life so you can understand how our caregivers' experiences influence our own. When I think of my mom, I picture her hands. I see her cutting and sautéing vegetables, mending clothes, or cleaning. Her hands have done more work in a decade than most people's do in a lifetime. I think, too, of the many times those hands held me or massaged my back. There were also times those hands were absent—unavailable to me when I needed them.

I remember how my mom shared tales of her unique childhood with me even before I started school. I learned how she and her family left Budapest, Hungary, in the back of an ambulance to flee a revolution. How they escaped Europe and were given refuge in Canada. How my grandpa wanted to settle his family in Washington, DC, but ended up in Washington State instead—all because of a language misunderstanding.

I remember feeling such awe for the adventures my mom had already experienced. For years, I was convinced that if she would teach me Hungarian, I would be unbelievably chic. But later I learned what it actually meant to be a refugee, to feel different. It meant loneliness when she couldn't speak English well and had to teach it to her parents. It meant being the only girl in her kindergarten with pierced ears. It meant trying to hide her accent from the jeers of her classmates and spending her childhood unlearning her native way of speaking.

Although as a kid I realized life had been hard for my mom, there was much about her story I didn't understand until I was older. I didn't realize how traumatic it was for her to grow up with an alcoholic father and a suicidal, depressed mother. I didn't realize how intensely she was affected by the death of her twin siblings in a house fire when she was seven, or the way that loss tinged her entire childhood with sadness and unspoken grief.

The more I learned about my mother, the more I understood how much she had to overcome and survive in her life.

Now I have a greater understanding as to why she turned to alcohol to cool the fierce aloneness she felt growing up—and all the ways she tried to self-medicate because of the intense dysfunction of her marriage. Though I've grieved it in layers over the last decade, I better understand why, though she loved me and my siblings fiercely, her own compounded trauma kept her triggered and at times unavailable when we needed her most. This was especially true when my father became unstable and his chaotic anger turned terrifying. We surely needed her then, but I see she was dealing with so much trauma that all her attempts to white-knuckle it couldn't stabilize the climate of our home.

My siblings and I paid a high price for living in a family like this. We never knew whether we would be praised or torn to shreds for a small mistake, and our sense of safety was stolen time and time again. I coped by trying to act as the adult when I was barely able to spell. I tried to be perfect, to ignore pain or suppress it until I was alone—living on constant high alert because it felt like the only way to manage the obstacle course of my life. Yet those coping skills could only get me so far—they couldn't help when the toxicity of my parents' marriage spilled over onto us.

My most vivid example of this happened the morning before my thirteenth birthday after a catastrophic argument between my parents the night before. I wondered what state our lives would be in as I walked down the creaky wooden stairs. The house felt different, empty. Typically, my mom woke way before us to get an early start on the day. But instead of seeing her coffee cup on the table or the warm light of the chandelier, I found only a short note saying that she loved us but couldn't stay anymore.

I had invited ten girls over for a slumber party the next day, but now I felt as if someone had thrown a heavy, wet blanket on me. I couldn't move; I simply ached, because where was my mom? Where was the parent I felt close to, whom I knew did the best she could to protect us? Was she okay? Was she hurt? Would I see her again?

Looking back, I don't know why my dad and I didn't cancel my slumber party. Instead, we acted as though everything were fine—my body found a way to white-knuckle through the gnawing pain. The girls came and went, and I have little memory of the sleepover. Mostly I recall feeling separate from and outside myself, all the while sensing that I had to hide the terrible secret of how broken my family really was, how fragmented I was. Even before my mom's breakdown and her self-medication with alcohol, and before my dad's emotional abuse became more frequent, some part of me knew things shouldn't be this way.

Inside, I was terrified. My mom—the one I had experienced as my safe parent—was gone, and I didn't know if she would ever return. Though I couldn't articulate it then, I feared she was dead. A week or so later, she did come back. Rumpled, gaunt, and exhausted, she looked as if she hadn't slept in weeks. She and my dad made an uneasy truce, and our lives progressed on unsteady ground.

My adolescence continued in this insecure fashion until it later crescendoed in my twenties with several addiction interventions with both parents. My mom chose to engage in treatment, and my dad chose to walk away from us. Ultimately it took discontinuing my relationship with him for me to truly begin to see just how harmful parts of my childhood had been.

Years of toxic stress had taken a toll on my body and soul in ways I couldn't yet understand. As I moved into adulthood, however, one thing seemed true: I felt more alone than ever. Theoretically, I knew I was loved by several people in my life, but I couldn't seem to hang on to that belief in a tangible way. Simply put, my body and soul had learned I couldn't depend on anyone, because they would *always* let me down or try to use me.

So as much as I *wanted* to trust people, the template I had internalized told me never to let my guard down. To the rest of the world, I appeared to be a strong, successful, driven person—after all, I was an honor roll student, a Christian, and a collegiate athlete. But on the inside, I felt scared. I felt alone. And I felt anxious.

HOW ATTACHMENT WORKS

Eventually, I would learn my relational fears were rooted in my earliest and ongoing relationships with my parents. Psychiatrist Curt Thompson explains that an infant

> will absorb his mother's anxiety simultaneously with the milk from her breast. He will distinguish the relative gentleness or roughness—or for that matter, the very presence or absence—of his father's physical

touch. He will notice the timing and intensity of his parents' responses to his pleasure as well as his distress. His brain will begin to register the general level of safety, tranquility, or chaos generated in the presence of each primary figure with whom he connects. . . . The nature of his relationships with his parents shapes the neural networks in a fashion that will have lifelong implications.[1]

These vital early experiences of responsiveness to our needs, which psychologists and researchers refer to as *attunement*, are the basis for our attachment styles throughout our lifespans.[2] Before any of us had even formed explicit thoughts or memories, the wiring in our brains and nervous systems began to mirror the ways our caregivers interacted with us—as well as how they responded when they purposefully or accidentally wounded us.[3] Even the most loving parents don't respond to their children perfectly,[4] which is why the concept of *repair* is vital. A repair occurs when caregivers recognize they've misattuned to their children and then figure out a way to reconnect, apologize, or take whatever step is needed. We now know this rupture/repair cycle can develop resilience. Yet it's not the wounding that breeds strength but the extent to which safety is reestablished by caregivers after moments of difficulty.[5] Resilience—or lack thereof—lies squarely in whether caregivers repair any breaches. The sum of these interactions with our caregivers lays the foundation for each of us to learn about ourselves and the world.

When a father assumes his baby wants to play peekaboo because of her wide-eyed gaze, he is rightly attempting to respond to what he believes is playfulness. Yet when he instead finds she's overstimulated and cranky, his ability to readjust his behavior to her needs is a form of repair.

When a mother snaps at her young son because he keeps interrupting her, he may cower in shame. But if the mom notices that her response has hurt him, she may stoop down to her little boy's level and gently say, "I'm so sorry I spoke that way to you. I felt frustrated by your interruption, but that doesn't make it okay." As the mom repairs the gap she created with her son, she becomes reattuned to his experience, and the son will move through the moment, confident once again in the security of his mom.

In my story, I didn't doubt my mom's love—but she was so caught up in her own pain that it was difficult for her to see all my bids for attention. Later my mom engaged in her own recovery, and she has done much to repair her connection with me as an adult. I still had to do my own work, but her willingness to honor my pain has allowed our relationship to grow, even with a difficult history. Now that I am an adult, my ability to heal isn't contingent on her repaired connection with me—because I can now tend to my wounds whether my parents choose to acknowledge them or not—but it has allowed us to have a much deeper relationship than I thought was possible.

When our childhood interactions with our caregivers are healthy—marked by attunement and consistent repair—they pave the way for us to feel safe, to learn how to regulate our emotions, to be willing to try new things, and to develop frameworks for future relationships.

So if you are a parent who is concerned about the ways you may be failing, my hope is you'll feel encouraged that this work doesn't demand perfection—just humility and awareness. Learning to try softer and cultivate self-awareness is a gift not only to ourselves but also to those we love. When parents are appropriately attentive and engaged with their kids because they themselves are connected to their own emotions, the children begin to develop an internal sense of self and form healthy relationships. Optimally, infants learn their caregivers are their "safe base" and that they have a soft place to land when life feels scary. Additionally, kids leverage this feeling of internalized safety as a way to help them explore the world, knowing they are free to be curious—because if they fall or experience difficulty, they can return to safety. This is what psychologists refer to as a secure attachment.

If at any point during development children experience untrustworthiness, disengagement, or abuse from their caregivers without appropriate repair, their attachment styles may be affected. No longer will these kids feel there is a safe shelter to return to, or a safe base from which to explore the world, and they may begin to adapt by white-knuckling through their experiences and relationships. The narrative that they must act okay, do it on their own, suppress their emotions, and sacrifice feeling safe just to be loved truly begins to take root. And because of that, they may be unable to try softer in their lives today.

ATTACHMENT STYLES AND YOU

Psychologist John Bowlby's pioneering work around attachment theory came to life when developmental psychologist Mary Ainsworth and her colleagues created the Strange Situation experiment in 1969.[6] In this study, children ages twelve to eighteen months were observed interacting with their mothers as well as complete strangers.

The experiment, which has been replicated many times, consisted of eight phases that lasted about three minutes each. First the infant and mother were ushered into a laboratory playroom, where they were invited to explore the room and its toys together. A stranger then joined them in the room. The stranger played with the baby while the mother left. The mother returned and the stranger exited. The mother left again, this time leaving the baby completely alone. The stranger returned and tried to comfort the baby. Finally, the mother returned and the stranger left.

As researchers observed consistent patterns of responses in the children, they developed several classifications for attachment—secure, anxious-ambivalent, avoidant, and later, disorganized. Each of these attachment styles describes how you—and your caregivers—may have experienced the world.

In the study, children who were *securely* attached appeared calm when a stranger joined them—as long as they were still in the company of their mothers. They experienced distress when their mothers left them alone with the stranger but were quickly soothed and calmed when the caregivers returned. Today, researchers believe that somewhere between 50 and 65 percent of Americans have a *secure* attachment style.[7] Those who carry secure attachment into adulthood typically experience greater success in relationships, adjust to difficulties more easily, and are able to draw upon better coping skills to self-soothe as necessary.

The children classified as having an *anxious-ambivalent* attachment style were equally distressed when their mothers left the room. However, these children displayed continued anxiety even *with* the returned presence of their mothers. Researchers theorized that the children acted this way because of their mothers' inconsistency or inability to accurately assess their children's emotional states. In other words, because the children with an anxious-ambivalent attachment didn't know whether their mothers would remain attentive and attuned to them, they remained anxious over the potential loss of that connection. This is not because of a flaw in the children; rather, their experiences with their mothers had wired their bodies to predict this. It is believed that 7 to 15 percent of Americans have an anxious-ambivalent style.[8] People with this type of attachment tend to struggle to directly state their needs to their partners, fear abandonment by those closest to them, and carry a belief that though others haven't disappointed them yet, they will.

A third group of children in the study demonstrated *avoidant* behavior; they appeared not to be fazed when their mothers left, by the presence of strangers, or when their mothers returned. Interestingly, while these children looked relaxed, their heart rates and internal responses were completely dys-regulated. In other words, while they appeared perfectly calm on the outside, their bodies were experiencing the situation as a crisis. Often children with this attachment style have experienced emotional frigidity and rejection from their parents, even though basic needs like food, shelter, and other physical necessities were provided. As a result, these children don't wonder whether their parents will be able to emotionally soothe them because they have already learned through experience that their parents won't. They have learned to isolate themselves to find calm, operating from a practical, emotionally distant, and self-reliant sphere as a way to disconnect from internalized feelings of rejection.

The final group of children in the study were those with a *disorganized* attachment, appearing to dissociate or become confused with the return of their mothers.[9] Rather than displaying the clear reactions of the other three types, these children showed elements of all three, though inconsistently. Children with this attachment style have typically experienced significant loss, trauma, or abuse. Because trauma overwhelms our systems and doesn't allow our bodies to process information correctly, these children didn't know how to react to their caregivers—they were the source of their trauma, and the kids had experienced them as terrifying and unpredictable in the past.

All of us tend to have a primary attachment style with those we are closest to; however, our attachment templates aren't static categories. Depending on who we are interacting with, our bodies may come to expect different responses.

For example, my primary attachment with my mom was an anxious-ambivalent style, although there were certainly some pieces of secure attachment too. My attachment style with my dad was largely disorganized with some anxious-ambivalent elements. Thus, I adapted to different situations and people using a mixture of all those lenses, depending on multiple factors. What's important to understand is that most of us will likely have some blending into other styles—and that's completely normal, even as we heal.

Safety and connection with our caregivers, it turns out, are critical to healthy human development and our relationships throughout life.

WHY THIS MATTERS FOR ADULTS

Interestingly, researchers found that almost all the parents of the children they were assessing in the Strange Situation experiment had the same attachment styles as their children. In general, the autonomous adults had been secure children; the preoccupied adults had been anxious-ambivalent children; the dismissive adults had been avoidant children; and the parents scarred by unresolved trauma or loss and/or caregivers they feared became dismissive adults. My mom couldn't help but give me the wounds she carried, because she had no idea there was a different way. This is how we all function. Like father, like son; like mother, like daughter. And so on.

Bottom line, if we cannot find ways to engage the work of repair from any unhealthy attachment style we developed as children, all of our later relationships will be greatly impacted. This isn't a life sentence; instead. it's an invitation to have compassion for our wounds so we can try differently in our relationships.

How might attachment styles play out in the life of Derek, who is waiting for his wife, Beth, to return home after spending an evening with friends? Beth said she would be home at about 7:00 to help with their kids' bedtime, but by 7:15, she hasn't arrived or called Derek.

Here's how the next few minutes will likely go, depending on Derek's attachment style:

If Derek has a secure attachment . . .

> Derek phones Beth: "Hey, honey, will you be home soon? I really need help with the kids tonight."
> Beth: "Yes, I'm so sorry. It'll probably be another ten minutes."
> Derek: "Okay, I know you didn't mean to get home late."

Derek may then be able to internally connect to the feeling that Beth is generally reliable and truly didn't mean to let him down. It's important to remember that a secure attachment doesn't mean perfection or complete self-sufficiency—instead it strikes the balance between independence and interdependence. Derek recognizes that he needs Beth, but he is able to sit with and attend to his own emotions when necessary.

If Derek has an anxious-ambivalent attachment . . .

> Derek calls Beth several times and finally reaches her
> at 7:30: "I can't believe you did it again. You never
> follow through on what you say."
> Beth: "Derek, I'm so sorry. But I haven't gotten home
> late in a long time."

Later Derek may struggle to let go of the anger he feels toward
Beth. After all, just as he predicted, she wasn't there when he
needed her. Derek may then feel as if he will need repeated
reassurances from Beth that she won't do this to him in the
future and she won't abandon him.

If Derek has an avoidant attachment . . .

Bedtime comes and goes, but Derek hasn't heard from Beth.
Derek's not angry; he just hadn't expected anything different.
If anything was going to get done, he would have to do it him-
self. It only confirmed what he'd always felt: He's on his own.

If Derek has a disorganized attachment . . .

It's 7:25, and Derek desperately wants to call Beth—but he
finds himself worried that if he calls her, she'll only get mad.
But he also worries that if she doesn't get home soon, he will
become overwhelmed and yell at the kids again. Derek feels as if
he is between a rock and a hard place. He suspects Beth means
well, but what if she later holds a grudge because he needed her?

ATTACHMENT STYLES

AUTONOMOUS

(Secure Attachment)

- *Tend to be interdependent and able to connect with others and themselves*
- *Can acknowledge their own faults while also hearing their partners' concerns*
- *Are able to stay emotionally regulated in everyday situations involving relationships*
- *Are able to more accurately assess whether a person is safe or reliable based on their previous experiences*

PREOCCUPIED

(Anxious-Ambivalent Attachment)

- *Tend to desire validation and closeness*
- *Are most afraid of abandonment*
- *Are hypercritical of self but more apt to see others as "good"*
- *Tend to be emotionally dysregulated when fearing relational disconnection*
- *Are typically triggered by conflict and react by wanting more closeness*
- *Experience the most engagement from their sympathetic nervous systems (fight/flight/fawn) when triggered[10]*

DISMISSIVE

(Avoidant Attachment)

- *Tend to be self-reliant*
- *Are most afraid of feeling "engulfed" by other people*
- *Tend to be critical of others but less critical of themselves*
- *Are emotionally disconnected*
- *Are typically triggered by conflict; react by isolating to try to emotionally self-regulate*
- *Experience the most engagement from their sympathetic nervous systems (fight/flight) when triggered[11]*

FEARFUL-AVOIDANT

(Disorganized Attachment)

- *Desire to connect to other people but also fear being used and hurt*
- *Are most afraid that those closest to them will cause them harm*
- *Tend to see themselves as defective and others as scary*
- *May feel they are inviting others in while also pushing them out*
- *Tend to be emotionally dysregulated, which may result in dissociation and/or sympathetic nervous system activation*
- *In relationships, may experience feelings reminiscent of the terror experienced in childhood*

Research confirms that we will likely project whatever attachment styles we adopt from our caregivers onto our relationship with God. In other words, folks who grew up with a safe attachment in their families will likely have a secure attachment style not only with other people but also with God.

When I recently reread some of my old journals from college, I recalled how badly I had wanted to please God and grow close to Him. I had wanted the abundant love He so generously offers us. What I understand now, though, is that part of my brain knew I was deeply loved by God, but because of my own unresolved trauma, I couldn't think myself into experiencing His love for me. Instead, I experienced Him as a tyrant, never pleased with anything I did. I longed to know Him as good; instead, I couldn't help but feel I was always in trouble—just waiting for the other shoe to drop. It's only been through intentionally working with my own pain that I have come to experience the true reality of a good, kind, and compassionate God.

HEALING INSECURE ATTACHMENT STYLES

If we grew up with an insecure attachment style, are we doomed? Can that be healed? Can we, too, experience God and others as safe? Thankfully, the answer is yes. Our internal working models *can* in fact be changed or repaired.

When this happens, it's referred to as *earned secure attachment*, which appears to happen in two steps.[12] First, we internalize a secure/autonomous attachment after developing a meaningful emotional relationship with a close friend, significant other, or therapist. Because of this nurturing connection, we are able to create a healthier "inner voice," one that sounds like the parent we needed—kind, gentle, compassionate. Using the prefrontal cortex, we can begin to observe where we feel wounded in areas of attachment and "reparent" them when we feel rejected, isolated, overly self-reliant, or scared. The second step occurs when we are able to coherently tell our story and understand from our own perspective why events happened.

What does that look like, you ask? Well, in my case, it happened like this: I had made plans to go to Denver and meet up with a friend from high school who had offered to host me as I interviewed for a nannying job. The last few months had been a roller coaster of unexpected events. In the span of six months after graduating from college, I'd become engaged, secured a job in banking, broken off the engagement, quit my

Ways to Talk to Your Inner Child (Reparenting)

- I'm listening.
- I'll set whatever boundaries are needed to help you feel safe.
- You're not alone anymore.
- I believe you.
- It's over now. Let's figure out a new way to be.

newly acquired job, moved to a different city, and moved home again. I assessed the damage and believed my life had thoroughly ended.

Emotionally, I was in a rocky place—to put it lightly. My trust in my own sense of direction and purpose had been lost after my relationship with my fiancé disintegrated. Our breakup reinforced my belief that I needed to perform to receive love. It also validated my belief that I wasn't enough, especially because I was part of a broken family and carried deep wounds.

And yet in the midst of my deep grief over what felt like numerous failures, I experienced a keen sense of God's presence with me. I listened and waited, and I felt prompted to do something outside my usual cautious nature: visit a city halfway across the country by myself to discern whether I should move there. What was I being called to do? I didn't know yet. I only knew this: God was asking me to risk. In the past, I had often felt I had too much to lose. This time, I knew I wanted God's peace and direction more than anything. My budding career and an entire season of life were over or ending, but I was willing to head to Denver if that was what it would take to gain a sense of wholeness. I finally had found a renewed sense of hope and purpose.

The last thing I thought I needed—or expected to do there—was to meet a man.

As I stepped off the plane at the Denver airport, all I saw were flat plains and an abundance of brown. September, I learned, is not a green season in Colorado. But more startling was the topography. *Where are all the mountains? Isn't this supposed to be the Mile High City?*

I met Brendan at a concert the day I arrived. My friend had set up a "chance" meeting between the two of us. My heart was raw, but he was kind, funny, and handsome, and a balm to my weary self. We hit it off immediately. Yet at certain times, unwelcome thoughts would intrude: I believed if Brendan truly knew my story—and me—he wouldn't like me, much less pursue a relationship with me. I felt sure I was too much. I felt, in some respects, unlovable, even though I wanted to be loved. I wanted Brendan to be with me, to care about me, to validate me. But I also tried to scare him off—all within a five-minute span of time.

Sounds pretty straightforward, right?

I gave my future husband a constant push and pull because I was afraid. I was terrified he would love me and leave me. I hid my fear with feigned self-confidence—sometimes I could even believe the best about myself. But always it came down to this truth: Growing up, I had experienced significant losses of trust in my parents, and this affected everything in my life. As our relationship developed, Brendan gave me hope that he could be a safe person by the ways he respected my boundaries, time, and energy—but my body was still catching up to what my mind, in part, already knew.

I didn't realize then that our wounds often surface only when at last we feel physically or emotionally safe. Once we are out of survival mode, our bodies, minds, and spirits can finally bear to consider our stories and the reasons we are so emotionally dysregulated.[13] In fact, it was just as we were settling into our new marriage that my feelings of insecurity and fear of abandonment became the worst. The logical part of my brain knew that Brendan was trustworthy, but that belief didn't seem to influence the anxiety that sat in the pit of my stomach.

Thankfully, we pursued counseling, and I discovered how chaos and trauma had affected my ability to connect with others. I learned that because of my early relationship with my parents, I had developed an insecure attachment style; more precisely, an anxious-ambivalent style with some disorganized qualities as well.

With this framework to understand the barriers we faced, I came to viscerally believe Brendan when he gave me his word. Instead of feeling that I needed to control him or that I was alone in the world, I experienced him as a place to be loved when I was weary. I came to believe Brendan held me in his heart as I held him in mine. And because he offered this love to me, I came to see that even when I wasn't with Brendan, I could offer this love to myself, too, through paying compassionate attention to my story. I had experienced *earned secure attachment.*

THE ULTIMATE ATTACHMENT

Though my earned secure attachment was birthed through my connection with my husband, these experiences of earned attachment can come in many different shapes and sizes.

We can experience this feeling of being known with friends, therapists, teachers, pastors, and even (and especially) God.

While there is no formulaic way for us to progress toward earned secure attachment with God or others, I can confidently say learning to try softer will help you better determine how to engage the journey. The work of paying compassionate attention is, in a sense, learning to steward for ourselves what God already believes about us—that we're valuable and loved. In a way, this work is about giving ourselves permission to receive the love that is available to us. It's less about "arriving" and more about paying attention to ourselves in the compassionate way we've always deserved.

Perhaps you've felt drawn to God for a long time. I was about six when I first felt the visceral sensation of knowing God was with me. And to my parents' credit—despite our chaotic home environment—they often talked with me about how I could know God. When I was a little older, I asked Jesus into my heart at every Billy Graham crusade and Christian basketball camp I attended. I wanted to be sure He knew how much I wanted and needed Him. Finding Him didn't take away my pain or the severe dysfunction in my home, but it did plant a seed of deep hope that I clung to with every ounce of strength I had.

Through His Word, Christ shows we have good reason to hold on to Him. Many times as I've worked on this particular chapter, I've found myself thinking about the parable of the Prodigal Son from Luke 15, which has become one of my favorite Scripture passages in the last few years. As

Scriptures for Building a Safe Attachment with God

"Even if the mountains walk away and the hills fall to pieces, my love won't walk away from you, my covenant commitment of peace won't fall apart." The GOD who has compassion on you says so.
ISAIAH 54:10, MSG

The LORD himself goes before you and will be with you; he will never leave you nor forsake you. Do not be afraid; do not be discouraged.
DEUTERONOMY 31:8, NIV

Whether or not your parents or caregivers provided you with a secure attachment, the passages above are just a few of the many places in Scripture where God invites you to rest in Him. As you read and meditate on the Scriptures below, allow yourself to experience the security, safety, and love that are yours in Christ.

Psalm 23 Ephesians 3:14-21
Psalm 34:4 Philippians 1:6
Psalm 61:1-2 Hebrews 10:23
Psalm 116:1-9 Hebrews 4:14-16
Romans 8:15 1 John 3:1

you may know, this is a tale Jesus told about two sons. The younger son asked his father for his inheritance and then left his family to spend it and live wildly; his older brother stayed home and continued to work for his father. Eventually, the younger son became weary of his wild life and ran out of money. He returned home, where—much to the consternation of his brother—he was lovingly welcomed back by their father.

It's easy to recognize that we all have elements of both sons in us. And just to be clear, I think that is an important part of the story. But these days, I keep coming back to the father and the way he lavished love on both sons. From an attachment perspective, the father acted as both a safe haven and a secure base for the wilder son:

He returned home to his father. And while he was still a long way off, his father saw him coming. Filled with love and compassion, he ran to his son, embraced him, and kissed him. His son said to him, "Father, I have sinned

64

against both heaven and you, and I am no longer worthy of being called your son."

But his father said to the servants, "Quick! Bring the finest robe in the house and put it on him. Get a ring for his finger and sandals for his feet. And kill the calf we have been fattening. We must celebrate with a feast, for this son of mine was dead and has now returned to life. He was lost, but now he is found." So the party began.

LUKE 15:20-24, NLT

The parable is striking, because from an attachment perspective, one of the primary aspects of who God is to us is a parent. And not just *any* parent—a good, kind, compassionate, stable, loving, and safe parent!

Notice the way the father in this parable attended to his son upon his return. He didn't shame him. There was no "I told you so." I'm sure the father knew the experience itself was enough of a teacher. What the son needed now was love and compassion so he could internalize the difficult lessons he had learned. In short, he needed the security of his father.

I particularly love how *THE MESSAGE* translation says that as the son apologized, "the father wasn't listening" (verse 22) because he was too busy preparing for the celebration. What a beautiful picture of the way God aches for us, receives us, and loves us. He is so set on loving and honoring us that instead of begrudgingly waiting for us to explain our behavior, He goes ahead and prepares a feast for us!

If feelings of rejection are a tender area in your life, too, can I invite you to let that sink in? Most of us do not expect to experience such grace from God after we've failed. We likely expect pain, or punishment, or shame. And to be sure, God doesn't always save us from the consequences of our actions. But He doesn't celebrate our pain either. He doesn't ask us to minimize it or pretend it isn't there. Instead, He offers His love and unending compassion as we walk through whatever we're facing.

Dear reader, this moves me so deeply. God is always on our side, providing comfort in ways that even our closest allies, friends, parents, and therapists cannot. Isaiah 49:15 provides yet another powerful picture of God as a parent: "Can a woman forget her nursing child, that she should have no compassion on the son of her womb? Even these may forget, yet I will not forget you." And in another parable, Jesus describes a man who has a hundred sheep and loses one. Jesus asks, "Doesn't he leave the ninety-nine in the open country and go after the lost sheep until he finds it?" (Luke 15:4, NIV).

Again and again He comes for us; He lovingly finds us. He makes a way where there was no way. As a Christian, this makes my heart rejoice. As a therapist, it makes me ecstatic. Like the missing puzzle piece that fits snugly and completes the pictures of our lives, God Himself is our best resource—the safest, best attachment we could ever have. And He is the only One who doesn't need to make repair attempts (although thank goodness the rest of us can make them when we blow it with one another).

You may not be fully experiencing God in this relational way yet, and that's okay. However, I hope you'll feel encouraged to know that the practice of trying softer is a way to integrate into your whole self what your brain, in part, may already know: You are phenomenally loved by the One who created you, so take heart. For those of us who did not experience what researcher Donald Winnicott called "good enough" parenting[14] and for those of us who struggle to find secure or reparative relationships in our lives right now, may we cling to the knowledge that our God is always with us.

TRY SOFTER

There is no question we were made for relationships; but they can be complicated, can't they? Is there an attachment style that stands out to you or feels true for you? Remember, most of us have more than one attachment style established by more than one caregiver. Typically, however, one style dominates how we relate to people. The questions below may help you identify your predominant style.

1. Take a moment to consider how you feel when you are near someone you would consider close to you. Do you feel calm? Anxious? Angry? Afraid?

2. Consider a person you would need to call if you were sick or hurting. If that person disappointed you in the past, think about how you reacted. Did you immediately withdraw? Did you tell them to

get away, but then immediately regret it and try to make amends? Did their actions make you feel disoriented or fearful?

3. Choose an affirmation below that will support you in trying softer with your wounds as you move toward an earned secure attachment.

   If you feel afraid that the people you need won't show up:
   I am loved no matter what—even when people mess up.

   If you tend to want to avoid connection when you are hurting:
   It's okay to ask for help. It's brave to ask for help.

   If you feel disconnected from yourself, others, and the moment:
   I am here, and it's okay to need connection.

4. Finally, if it feels comfortable to do so, invite God into your experience. If the story of the Prodigal Son feels nurturing, take a moment and use it as a template to experience God welcoming you. Allow yourself to hear the words and feel the compassion that God lavishes on His children through this story.

   What do you see in this image?
   What do you hear?
   What do you smell?
   Tune in to what your body is telling you by noticing any sensations you feel.
   Where do you notice them? As you feel more connected to the image you are thinking about, breathe and simply let yourself be with this nurturing image.

For now, simply notice that you may lead with a certain attachment style, and give yourself permission to honor this. At some point, preferably with a therapist or another trusted person, spend time sharing about your experiences with this exercise.

If you are one of the nearly 35 to 50 percent of Americans who struggle with insecure attachment, take heart in knowing that becoming aware of it is a significant stride toward healing. The way we unlearn and heal our wounded attachment styles is by experiencing safe relationships, leaning into them, and then utilizing those felt experiences of care to reshape how we see ourselves and others.

WE ARE NOT

DEFINED BY

OUR BEST DAYS OR

OUR WORST DAYS.

WE ARE HIS

BELOVED.

CHAPTER 4

TOO HOT, TOO COLD . . . JUST RIGHT:

FINDING YOUR WINDOW OF TOLERANCE

She had not known the weight, until she felt the freedom!
NATHANIEL HAWTHORNE, *The Scarlet Letter*

REMEMBER THE FAIRY TALE featuring Goldilocks? As a family of bears takes a walk through the forest while their breakfast porridge cools, this fair-haired little girl enters their house and begins to look around. She eats the bowl of cereal that is neither too hot nor too cold; sits on and breaks the chair that is neither too big nor too small; and finally falls asleep in the bed that is neither too hard nor too soft. Though parents and teachers have assigned a number of morals to this story, I like how trauma therapist Deb Dana considers it through the lens of emotional arousal: Essentially, when it comes to the ability to sit with our feelings and experiences, each of us has a range that feels "just right." She refers to this as "the Goldilocks principle."[1]

And just as one version of the fairy tale has Goldilocks

jumping out of the window when the unhappy bears found her in one of their beds, so we often become overwhelmed and act without thinking when our nervous systems have been triggered by real or perceived threats. We call this moving outside our window of tolerance.

We've talked about the impact of trauma and the importance of experiencing our caregivers as safe and attentive. If we didn't have that experience—and especially if our stories include toxic stress or distressing events—our ability to tolerate discomfort lessens, and we more easily go into *hyper*arousal (fight/flight/fawn) or *hypo*arousal (freeze/dissociation). Additionally, our window of tolerance may be affected by medical issues, physiology, or ongoing adverse conditions. These states of hyper- and hypoarousal occur on a spectrum, with their accompanying thoughts, emotions, and bodily sensations intensifying depending on how far outside of our comfort levels we get.

The space between hyper- and hypoarousal, what might be thought of as the "just right" amount of intensity, is the range in which we can experience emotions, sensations, and experiences without feeling physiologically overwhelmed. First named by Dr. Daniel Siegel but additionally strengthened through the work of Dr. Stephen Porges, this range is our *window of tolerance* (WOT).[2] Each of us has a WOT, whether we find we are constantly pushing against the edges of it or not. When we are in our window, the brain stays integrated with the prefrontal cortex, which allows us to pay compassionate attention to ourselves and to try softer. This is where we want to be.

The events that push people out of their WOT vary. Take Erin, for example—a sleep-deprived fifteen-year-old. Though her parents love her, she feels she can never show weakness academically, so she stays awake late into the night to finish her homework. One day at lunch, she notices the two most popular girls in her grade laughing at her. Immediately Erin's heart starts racing, and she runs out of the cafeteria. She was already so physically and emotionally run-down that she left her WOT as soon as she saw the girls smirking at her.

Or think of Collette, who recently experienced a miscarriage and feels unsure of how to process her loss. While in traffic, someone cuts her off. Without thinking, she begins to

When I'm in HYPERAROUSAL (fight/flight/fawn), I may feel:	When I'm in my WINDOW OF TOLERANCE, I may feel:	When I'm in HYPOAROUSAL (freeze), I may feel:
• overwhelmed with adrenaline; • my heart racing; • physical shaking/trembling; • the urge to move my body—either away from or toward the stressful event; • angry; • out of control; • scared; • anxious; or • the need to overaccommodate or to please people.	• strong; • competent; • curious; • relaxed; • content; • balanced; • able to rationally make decisions; • hopeful; or • able to take risks without feeling overwhelmed.	• sluggish; • depressed; • suddenly exhausted; • foggy/zoned out; • paralyzed—frozen to the spot; • numb/shut down; • disconnected from the world; or • as though I'm watching myself.

shout angry comments she never thought would come out of her mouth. She, too, is finding herself outside her window.

Finally, there is Ray, who grew up hearing the phrase "Boys don't cry." After he loses his dream job over a series of unavoidable issues, he finds himself checked out in front of the television for hours at a time. His nervous system is overwhelmed, and the weight of his sadness has plunged him out of his window and into hypoarousal.

Each of these examples shows us that sometimes when difficulties compound, what we once felt we could handle begins to feel unbearable. Even everyday experiences can add up and make us less able to navigate unpleasant situations, pushing us out of our WOT.

The good news is this: Though our windows of tolerance are different in size, they can all be widened over time, bringing great benefits:

- Rather than responding to perceived threats by automatically moving into fight/flight/fawn or freeze, we are able to draw on the natural ability of our bodies to process and move through difficult experiences.
- We are better equipped to heal from past trauma.
- Once we understand the limits of our tolerance and how to stay within them, we can try softer, working with our bodies to mindfully push through and increase those limits.

No matter how much we long to change, we need to be mindful of our WOT before confronting fears or difficulties. Trying to white-knuckle or shame ourselves into expanding our limits before we're ready can actually backfire. Consider Jen, who arrived at my office for the first time breathless and apologetic. We quickly developed a strong rapport, and I could sense her commitment to addressing several destructive patterns in her life. She spoke of verbally abusive relationships, body shame, and a self-critic that didn't quit.

When we discussed her childhood, Jen told me of the many times her father had promised to take her somewhere special, only to arrive home drunk and verbally abusive. These childhood wounds significantly affected her adult relationships and the way she learned to exist in the world—she always doubted the love of the people closest to her and never felt at rest.

She had tried counseling once before, but after two months of meeting regularly with her therapist, she'd become so overwhelmed by anxiety attacks that she stopped going. She reached out to me after hearing me speak about trauma-informed therapy. Early on, Jen told me she was still dead set on working through her issues as quickly as possible. She said, "I know this whole trauma-informed perspective puts a high value on feeling safe, but I just want to muscle through all this stuff, you know?"

I was grateful that Jen felt she could be honest, because it allowed me to help her understand my approach—one that would enable her to remain in her WOT as she developed the resources that would help her work through her experiences rather than be flooded by them.

I could tell that Jen's previous counselor had cared deeply about her, but as we explored why Jen had stopped seeing her, it became clear that they had moved too fast—jumping right into areas of her life that Jen wasn't ready to handle. Like a bodybuilder who suddenly attempts to triple the amount of weight he can lift, Jen had overwhelmed and further wounded her nervous system by trying to move toward healing too quickly. Afraid she'd be judged if she talked to her counselor about her heightened anxiety, Jen simply quit counseling. After a few months of feeling that all she could do was survive—barely—she finally reached out to me.

Jen's experience is precisely why I move carefully and provide as many psychological resources as I can to help clients move slowly but purposefully toward living awake rather than feeling overwhelmed or numb—far outside their WOT.

Put another way, once Jen learned how to stay in her WOT even when triggered, she enabled her mind and body to reintegrate parts of her story that had been too painful to deal with, which meant she finally had a cohesive life narrative. Additionally, Jen came to understand that as she learned and respected the interior of her own WOT, she was actually taking a step toward healing, because she was listening to what she needed rather than having others dictate it to her. In this way, she was trying softer.

WHAT MOVES US IN AND OUT OF THE WINDOW

As we work to recognize our own WOT, it's important to understand what is driving our bodies to move in and out of them. Researchers are just beginning to understand how the *vagus* nerve influences our responses in different emotional states. The vagus is the longest cranial nerve in the body, running from the brain into the face and ears and then down to major organs in the chest and abdomen, including the heart, lungs, intestines, and stomach.[3] One section of this nerve is responsible for enabling us to stay in our WOT. This section is called the *ventral vagal complex* and controls the social engagement system, and it's what most people use (unconsciously, of course!) when they want to connect with others or relax.

A far less advanced section of the vagus nerve is called the *dorsal vagal complex*. It is what plunges our bodies into disconnection or dissociation (hypoarousal), and similar to what happens in hyperarousal, the top of the brain goes offline. However, this doesn't just happen randomly. Essentially, scientists have discovered that if something activates our nervous systems, there is a particular order in which our bodies respond to threats. They react involuntarily based on our attachment styles, physiology, and life experiences.

For example, let's say you and a team from work are enjoying a leisurely afternoon retreat at a coworker's house when you suddenly hear a loud bang that alarms you. If you are in your WOT, you will likely look around to see if someone can help. You make eye contact with your coworker and ask her what the sound was. She explains that someone upstairs was closing a door that needs fixing. This interaction helps your body know that you're not alone and that the sound did not signal danger. As a result, you are able to "digest" the emotional intensity that came up when you were startled. This is an example of using your social engagement system (ventral vagal) and staying in your WOT.

Let's imagine a second scenario that takes place in the

SYMPATHETIC NERVOUS SYSTEM	VENTRAL VAGAL SYSTEM	DORSAL VAGAL SYSTEM
(tend to access first in crisis)		(tend to access after sympathetic nervous system doesn't resolve threat)
When I'm in HYPERAROUSAL (fight/flight/fawn), I may feel:	When I'm in my WINDOW OF TOLERANCE, I may feel:	When I'm in HYPOAROUSAL (freeze) I may feel:
• overwhelmed with adrenaline;	• strong;	• sluggish;
• my heart racing;	• competent;	• depressed;
• physical shaking/ trembling;	• curious;	• suddenly exhausted;
• the urge to move my body—either away from or toward the stressful event;	• relaxed;	• foggy/zoned out;
	• content;	• paralyzed—frozen to the spot;
	• balanced;	• numb/shut down;
• angry;	• able to rationally make decisions;	• disconnected from the world; or
• out of control;	• hopeful; or	• as though I'm watching myself.
• scared;	• able to take risks without feeling overwhelmed.	
• anxious; or		
• the need to overaccommodate or to please people.		

same setting—an afternoon retreat at your coworker's house. This time, however, you are already nearing the edge of your WOT after a difficult week—you don't feel close to anyone at the gathering, and because of the chaotic narrative of your life, you feel too vulnerable to ask for help when the loud bang occurs. You also don't yet have a strong sense of how to comfort yourself when you're overwhelmed. You look around after the loud bang but don't see anyone you think could help ease your fear. And then because of past traumas, your neurobiology takes over. It's likely your sympathetic nervous system will quickly shoot you into fight-or-flight mode. Perhaps you come up with a hasty excuse to leave immediately. Or maybe you simply feel agitated and can't focus on what people are saying to you. For the rest of the meeting, you may feel off, knowing everything is probably fine but lacking a way to help yourself regulate.

Now, if you have a history of experiencing certain types of trauma, your response to a banging door is likely to be even more extreme. Although the sound of the banging door is not necessarily dangerous, your coping strategy tells you that shutting down is the safest way to deal with this possible threat, and you will likely bypass your social engagement system (i.e., ignore the instinct to reach out for help), perhaps only briefly experience the urgency of fight/flight, and then move right into dissociation (the dorsal vagal complex). This can feel like fogginess, disconnection, immobilization, fainting, or a complete loss of awareness of time. These types of responses occur because the most primitive part of the vagus nerve has been activated, and your body concludes there is no escape.[4] Again, it's important to remember that this isn't a conscious decision; rather, it is your body's best attempt to neutralize what it believes to be a threat. Later, you may not remember many details of the retreat, or you may possibly feel as though you were disconnected the whole time—as though you were "there, but not there."[5]

I share these possible scenarios with you for a couple of reasons. First, many of us have deep shame around our feelings of anxiety or disconnection—as if we should be stronger than we are, or just "get over" our fears. But what I want you to hear is this: It's important that we honor our stories, and it's vital that we understand and have compassion for the biological responses our bodies now have because of those stories. Many of these responses happen whether we want them to or not.

Second, when we understand the physiology of our bodies, we can be empowered to try softer with ourselves. If trying softer means remaining aware and engaged with our bodies, we will ultimately strengthen our ability to stay in our WOT.

If you grew up without a secure attachment, you may not feel you can reach out for help when scared—this is a clue that your experiences have made your WOT smaller. But you don't have to stay there, my friends. Once you begin to learn to connect safely with others—which is part of learning to try softer—the social engagement system will help keep you regulated and calm. In our "afternoon retreat" scenario, all it might take is reaching out to a coworker for connection, reaffirming to your body that you are safe, and using any tools needed to keep you in your WOT.

Trying softer allows us to recognize that we must figure out how to establish safety for our bodies. If we can listen to and respond to our bodies' needs, whether that means releasing energy by getting outside or staying connected to ourselves through conscious breathing, our WOT will begin to grow, and true healing can occur. It is slow work, but friend, nothing could be more worth it.

CREATING A NEW FRAMEWORK

As we've seen, our earliest core relationships not only dictate our attachment styles but also help determine the size of our WOT. And as we do the work of digging into and honoring our stories, we begin to gain insight into *why* we struggle to stay in our WOT. As Dr. Daniel Siegel writes, "The mind we first see in our development is the internal state of our caregiver. . . . So we first know ourselves as reflected in the other."[6]

For example, a baby whose mother mirrors a sad face back to him when he is crying will come to understand that her expression reflected his own feeling of sadness or distress. Ideally, as the baby grows toward adulthood, he'll build on these experiences of care to attend to his own feelings, even if someone else isn't there. If we've been given developmental support, we come to know instinctively how to pay compassionate attention to ourselves.

But if we are parents with our own trauma histories or if we never learned how to feel our own feelings, we cannot model doing so to our children unless we, too, learn to regulate our own emotions. For example, if as children we were shamed anytime we felt pain, we may become angry when our preschooler stubs her toe and cries profusely instead of providing connection and compassion to help her move through the pain. If we never have the opportunity to practice feeling our emotions in the presence of another person's more grounded nervous system, our WOT remains very small, and we are more likely to become emotionally dysregulated quickly.

When I began dating Brendan, I initially was overwhelmed by the possibility that someone could be consistent enough in their care for me that I could trust them. I had lived in a state of almost constant hyperarousal for much of my life because I needed to be able to react quickly to the chaos and unpredictability of my family—I had a small WOT and was used to living way outside it. As I mentioned in chapter 3, I did come to trust Brendan. Over time, I was also able to relate to God, other people, and myself differently. This made space for me to listen to my body and prepared me to understand what trying softer might look like when my counseling supervisor invited me to approach my life in this way.

SEEING GOD IN THE WINDOW

A few years ago during the holiday season, I was sitting in our quiet living room after our daughter, Matia, had fallen asleep.

Christmas lights twinkled on the tree, and I exhaled a sigh of relief as I thought back on our grand night. We'd gone ice-skating, sipped hot chocolate, and then taken a drive through the neighborhood to look at lights. After Brendan and I had spent extra time with Matia on bedtime wrangling, kisses, and tuck-ins, my husband ran out to pick up a few things from the grocery store. I finally had time to sit, and since becoming a mom, I had come to savor this time—when all was finally quiet.

Matia had had a ball that night to be sure, but as I sat on the couch, I realized how sad I felt, right alongside my happy. I wanted to connect only with the bright spots like this in my life, but I knew those parts of my story were intertwined with painful pieces. As I sat there, I realized that in order to feel the good, I also needed to acknowledge the hard. This, I was learning, is part of what it means to try softer; it requires listening to what is actually going on inside of me.

I sat wrapped in my favorite blanket, with my legs crisscrossed, and tried to embrace with compassion the myriad of emotions I was experiencing. I realized holidays had often brought waves of grief for me. My young self had experienced years of heartache, crushed expectations, and days that should have been joyous but instead were mired with pain.

Yet on this night I began to notice something new in this place of ache: a sense of God's nearness with me as I considered my story—and not simply in a logical way. I also felt His presence in a physical way.

What God Says about His Beloved

Because he bends down to listen, I will pray as long as I have breath!
PSALM 116:2, NLT

You are so intimately aware of me, Lord. You read my heart like an open book and you know all the words I'm about to speak before I even start a sentence! You know every step I will take before my journey even begins. You've gone into my future to prepare the way, and in kindness you follow behind me to spare me from the harm of my past. With your hand of love upon my life, you impart a blessing to me.
PSALM 139:3-5, TPT

The LORD appeared to us in the past, saying: "I have loved you with an everlasting love; I have drawn you with unfailing kindness."
JEREMIAH 31:3, NIV

The lights on the tree cast a soft glow as I looked down at my hands, and for a moment, I simply felt held. I sensed it then, as surely as I know my own name—God with me: Emmanuel, the One whom I had loved since my elementary school days, had become more than words I'd read or some far-off hope. Our small living room became a bit of a sanctuary, and I sat with the presence of the One who loves me so. I breathed in a sacredness I had felt only intermittently in my life and could never quite hold on to. I realized I still felt sad, but I didn't feel alone.

In this precious moment, I was able to recognize how my own WOT had grown precisely because of how I moved through feelings of discomfort that bubbled up.

And even more importantly, in this moment I experienced God as a secure attachment in the same way I had come to experience Brendan as secure. I had not worked my way into this, had not hustled or tried hard to experience God; instead, God came near when I was open—to Him, to the truth about myself, and even to Brendan.

I cannot tell you what this meant to me. In the previous few years, my husband and I had been struggling with secondary infertility. My dashed hopes of building our family felt raw and tender. This season of unmet desire had reminded me of my own doubt in God's love. I kept trying to white-knuckle myself out of the grief, but it wasn't working.

I wanted to believe God is good, but the time of waiting and asking and yet not receiving caused me to wonder, *How does God feel about my pain? My heartache? Is He truly safe, as I had thought and hoped? Or has it been a sham?*

Is He trying to punish me because I am not enough? Or does He grieve over the things that hurt me too?

As I honestly contemplated these questions in this space with God, I began to weep. Though He gave me no answers that night, His loving presence reassured me that I was safe with Jesus. It became okay not to know. Gradually my breathing slowed, my shoulders relaxed, and I

Are you tired? Worn out? Burned out on religion? Come to me. Get away with me and you'll recover your life. I'll show you how to take a real rest. Walk with me and work with me— watch how I do it. Learn the unforced rhythms of grace. I won't lay anything heavy or ill-fitting on you. Keep company with me and you'll learn to live freely and lightly.
MATTHEW 11:28-30, MSG

I am convinced that neither death nor life, neither angels nor demons, neither the present nor the future, nor any powers, neither height nor depth, nor anything else in all creation, will be able to separate us from the love of God that is in Christ Jesus our Lord.
ROMANS 8:38-39, NIV

could sit with all the pieces of my life—good and bad—knowing God was there and I was profoundly loved.

BELOVED

We didn't get to choose the dynamics of our childhood or ask for the relational wounds we may have experienced. This is one reason I love to teach people about their WOT, their bodies, and how God will walk beside them on their journeys. We have the power to change our futures.

One of the best parts of learning to open myself up to God and allowing Him to sit with me in my joy and grief is this: I have learned to see myself as He sees me. God has many beautiful names for each of us, but one that came out of the season where I reexperienced God as safe is *Beloved*. This term has become sacred to me because it represents the connectedness and growth that have allowed me to try softer in life. It reminds me that God is the most loving, tender parent I could have.

Years ago, I picked up Henri Nouwen's book *Life of the Beloved*, and it changed the trajectory of my thinking about my own identity. Nouwen challenges readers to see themselves as united with the identity of Jesus. In Mark 1, John baptizes Jesus, and then a voice from heaven says, "You are my beloved Son; with you I am well pleased" (verse 11). As my friend Karen González notes, "God affirmed Jesus' value even before he had accomplished a thing in his earthly ministry."[7] Or as we think of ourselves as God's beloved, perhaps we could borrow from the relationship between Jesus and John, "the disciple whom Jesus loved" (John 21:20).

I wonder what it would be like for you to imagine that God thinks of you in this way. No matter how your day goes, what you do or don't accomplish, where you fail or succeed, or how scared or overwhelmed you might feel, you would know He is the One who lovingly watches out for you, who is delighted just to be near you. That's the goodness embedded in your very existence, dear reader.

During our hardest, scariest times—whether our bodies feel stressed and jumpy or sluggish and slow—God is there to reassure us that we are not defined by our best days or our worst days. We are His beloved.

TRY SOFTER

Containment

As we seek to honor or expand our WOT, we sometimes need additional support when we're feeling especially triggered or when something is especially hard. A strategy we can use to feel some healthy distance from the trigger is called *containment*. We can use this exercise to give our nervous systems a break when we have uncomfortable experiences or sensations so we can come back to them when we choose to rather than feeling trapped as they are happening to us.[8]

1. Picture something that feels strong enough to hold your internal disturbance. You can choose whatever you want; many folks visualize a treasure chest with chains around it, a strong safe, or even the hands of God holding the disturbance for them. Take a moment to be creative and choose something that allows your body to feel relief, knowing you can come back to the underlying issue at any time.

2. Once you've chosen a container, visualize putting the disturbing content inside it. Take as much time as you need. If you sense the container is not strong enough to hold the content, consider adding a second layer of protection between the container and you. For example, picture taking a safe that's wrapped up in chains and shoving it to the bottom of the ocean.

3. Once the disturbance is contained, consider moving into the following breath prayer.

Breath Prayer

Research shows that taking longer to exhale than to inhale signals to our nervous systems that we are safe, stimulating the vagus nerve.[9] Both help us stay in our WOT.

You can also incorporate a breath prayer to anchor you and support you as you breathe. I love the simplicity and significance of another name God uses for Himself, *Yahweh*, which is rooted in the Hebrew letters that compose the phrase "I AM" (Exodus 3:14). We know that out of reverence, speaking the name of Yahweh became taboo for the Jewish people at some point, yet Richard Rohr notes that it seems to mimic our very breath: "The one thing we do every moment of our lives is . . . to speak the name of God. This makes it our first and last word as we enter and leave the world."[10]

To practice the breath prayer,

1. Choose *Yahweh* or another two-syllable word to anchor you.

2. Inhale through the nose with *Yah* (or the first syllable) for three seconds.

3. Exhale with *weh* through the mouth (or the second syllable) for six seconds.

As you feel able, practice this conscious breathing for one to two minutes.

THE WORK OF
BOUNDARIES
BEGINS WITH
OUR BODIES.

CHAPTER 5

BOUNDARIES BRING US LIFE

You are not required to set yourself
on fire to keep other people warm.
UNKNOWN

"I KNOW THAT IT SHOULDN'T BE SO HARD to let people down,"
Anya said, "but it's soooo difficult."

During our session, she explained why she was sure she
was about to disappoint her mother, whom she knew would
not take it well. Her eyes welled up with tears as she spoke.

"I know exactly what I need to do. Truly. It's not hard. But
every time I start to tell my mom that I can't host our family
Thanksgiving, she cuts me off and reminds me that it would
be her only chance to be with her seven grandkids this year.
And then my heart races out of my chest. All of a sudden,
I feel like I'm a little kid again," she told me.

Those who know Anya might find this conversation odd.
She seems so accomplished and well-spoken, and she enjoys

spending time with her extended family. Yet she had recently gone back to work full time after her youngest started school, and because of her new responsibilities, she just didn't feel she could invite people to her home for the holidays.

Anya shared that, of course, some part of her knows life includes having to disappoint people—but for much of her childhood she had learned that she didn't actually have the right to say no. "Those weren't the words communicated to me exactly," she said. Instead, she picked up the message through nonverbal cues.[1] Her parents simply modeled and confirmed over and over again that she didn't have a choice or a voice.

Once when she was ten, Anya did try to advocate for herself when she felt her teacher had unfairly criticized her in front of the entire class. Instead of supporting her, Anya's parents banned her from participating in extracurricular activities for a month. They made her feel searing shame for embarrassing them by standing up to her teacher. Anya told me that her mom never would have told her own mother or husband no, and whenever Anya's preference didn't match that of her parents, she was either belittled or scolded. The discomfort Anya felt afterward seemed worse than simply going along with whatever they wanted.

What Anya shared with me is representative of my own experiences, as well as those of many of my clients. For kids who grow up with insecure attachments and lots of little t trauma, trying to understand the rules is a never-ending process—one that can last well into adulthood. *If I make a mistake, will I be raged at or quickly forgiven? Is it okay to ask people to stop yelling at me? At others? Is it possible that my opinion could be as valid as theirs?*

Maybe you've struggled with similar questions: *If my dad said yes, did he actually mean it? Or would he later deny saying it and pin the misunderstanding on me? If I tried to understand the pattern, would I feel as if I were just banging my head against the wall, because there was no pattern?*

When our caregivers continually communicate that we don't have a voice, we may learn it's better just to tell them what they want to hear. Then we carry that perception into adulthood and our relationships with other people. Rather than going into fight or flight during hyperarousal, we may channel that energy into overaccommodating others as a way to neutralize a perceived threat. Just like all responses to trauma, much of this happens on a subconscious level. The main goal of our bodies is to keep us safe, and the fawn response (which was introduced in chapter 2) is a learned reaction to the belief that it's better to stay "safe" than to ruffle feathers. When this is the script we live from, we are likely to mistrust our own instincts and avoid advocating for ourselves. Additionally, our window of tolerance is narrow because we've constantly had to deny or suppress our own emotions in order to keep others happy, which makes us less able to manage whatever life throws at us. It also can make learning to try softer more difficult since we've had to become overly attuned to the demands of others as a way to exist in the world. As a result, we have little practice listening to our own experiences.

As Anya and I talked more about her mom's demand that she host Thanksgiving, I helped her pay attention to what her body was telling her. She noticed that her breathing was shallow and that her shoulders felt tight—simply imagining a conversation in which she would tell her mom she couldn't host the dinner made her anxious and uptight. (To get her out of her head, I also walked her through a grounding exercise to bring her focus back to the present moment. You'll learn more about this technique on page 111.) Clearly Anya's belief that she couldn't set limits with her mother had driven her out of her WOT.

Anya—like many of us—learned early on that setting a limit with anyone, especially someone you care about, is disrespectful, and that being a "good Christian" means you have to give people what they want, no matter what. But this isn't true. Jesus, who showed us how to fully embrace our finite, beloved humanity, often said no, communicated His preferences, and set limits:

> Before daybreak the next morning, Jesus got up and went out to an isolated place to pray. Later Simon and the others went out to find him. When they found him, they said, "Everyone is looking for you."
>
> But Jesus replied, "We must go on to other towns as well, and I will preach to them, too. That is why I came."
>
> MARK 1:35-38, NLT

I have no right to say who will sit on my right or my
left. God has prepared those places for the ones he
has chosen.

MARK 10:40, NLT

One day some parents brought their children to
Jesus so he could lay his hands on them and pray
for them. But the disciples scolded the parents for
bothering him.

But Jesus said, "Let the children come to me.
Don't stop them! For the Kingdom of Heaven
belongs to those who are like these children."

MATTHEW 19:13-14, NLT

Don't waste what is holy on people who are unholy.
Don't throw your pearls to pigs! They will trample
the pearls, then turn and attack you.

MATTHEW 7:6, NLT

Jesus was ultimately a suffering servant, but He lived
out this truth from a place of choice—not because He was
shamed into it. Read that again. He invites *us* to live from
this place of freedom too. When we do, we may realize that
the stories imprinted on our brains may feel real but are not
necessarily true anymore.

Certainly, the Bible shows us that God absolutely hardwired us for connection. But through Jesus, we see that we

were also made to become our own selves—to be inter-dependent, not completely dependent on or avoidant of each other. And if our caregivers didn't give us the tools to develop our attachments appropriately, we can be hindered from doing what God made us for. This idea of remaining connected and interdependent (but not dependent) is deeply biblical.

In their book *Boundaries,*[2] Henry Cloud and John Townsend discuss the difference between bearing each other's burdens and carrying our own loads. This concept comes from Galatians 6:

> Bear one another's burdens, and so fulfill the law of Christ. For if anyone thinks he is something, when he is nothing, he deceives himself. But let each one test his own work, and then his reason to boast will be in himself alone and not in his neighbor. For each will have to bear his own load.
>
> VERSES 2-5

This passage reminds us that some things in life are too big to handle alone, while other tasks truly are ours to handle individually. Boundaries are necessary when someone asks us to handle their "load." Many clients I work with grew up in families where they were required to take on other people's individual loads but weren't permitted to ask for help with their legitimate burdens.

How might this play out? Parents may try to make their children into little adults by sharing mature information, emotions, or situations and expecting the children to "handle" it for them. Perhaps a mother overshares with her ten-year-old son about her marital issues, or a father repeatedly talks to his children about the family's financial woes. These types of interactions are hurtful to children because they don't yet have the emotional resources to process what the adults are asking of them—yet the kids may feel they have no choice but to try. Alternately, when these same children feel overwhelmed by trying to process all the adult content they've been given, they may be belittled for asking for support.

Perhaps you can see how all this can affect us even into adulthood. Instead of living with healthy interdependence so we can voice our limits and needs, we may have learned that our needs are always less valid than those of others.

We all have the ability to ask for help with our burdens—and we should—but when someone commands us to do

Simple Ways to State a Boundary

1. "Thanks so much for asking, but I'm not available."
2. "Sorry, that won't work for me."
3. "I'm not comfortable with that—I think I'll pass."
4. "You can handle it however works best for you, but count me out."
5. "No."

something, it is different from them asking for assistance. In healthy adult relationships, we flex and bend with one another as we recognize that all of us are finite and that often, even when people want to, they can't meet all our needs. If we were taught that it is normal to arrange our preferences and schedules around our families' or to conform to authority figures' whims when they are angry, that is the narrative that has kept our bodies in a hypervigilant state. And that isn't a narrative God wants for us, my friend.

Setting boundaries is complex, difficult work, but I promise that as we begin to set limits and learn to listen to what our bodies are telling us, we will start experiencing the freedom that comes with hearing the heartbeat of our internal world. This is part of the foundation that will help us thrive.

THERE'S A REASON WE DON'T SET LIMITS

Like everything in this book, the work of boundaries begins with our bodies. While most of us realize conceptually that it's okay to set boundaries, the feelings of dread, anxiety, and shame that come with disappointing people often keep us from doing so. As we've seen, this is often—though not always—tied to a childhood narrative that taught us that if we didn't do what was expected, we might face intolerable consequences. Our minds have stored these thoughts as implicit memories, subconscious understandings that inform our later perceptions of situations or that cause us to repeat actions without thinking about them.

But what does this actually mean? If you can drive a car, or chew gum and walk at the same time, or put your keys back in the drawer without remembering you did it, you do so because of implicit memory. Similarly, when you smell your grandma's cookies and feel comforted, or when you always expect bad news when the phone rings, this is also because of implicit memory. There are things you just know in the deepest parts of you.

As with attachment, watching our caregivers set their own limits engages the mirror neurons in our brains, thereby creating templates in our implicit memories for us to follow. Mirror neurons work like predictive text on our phones—automatically filling in what they think we'll type next based on our previous texts. In the same way, mirror neurons tell our brains how something is supposed to go based on our previous experiences.[3]

Mirror neurons also help us develop empathy for other people's experiences, as well as our own. For example, if three-year-old Max and his mom are playing with blocks and Max suddenly smacks her on the cheek, his mom may say, "Ouch. That hurt me. I want to play with you, but not if you hit. We'll have to take a break from this and calm down because it's not okay to hit other people." His mom is setting a limit with Max and giving him the opportunity to observe her pain, and the whole experience adds to his template the fact that there are times to say no. Later when Max goes to a friend's house and his friend hits him, Max may say, "Ouch. I want to play with you, but not if you hit me." After a childhood with these types of interactions, Max will hopefully grow into an adult who knows it's okay to say no, and he will also expect that sometimes people will say no to him.

Over time, as we observe how different relational contexts cause pain or discomfort, our bodies pull from our existing templates to help us know how to handle them. The way our caregivers treated us, themselves, and others is what helps us understand the bigger picture of boundaries.

Of course, our caregivers can also teach the opposite. If our limits aren't respected and our opinions aren't valued, our brains sense danger and often become triggered. As we discussed in chapter 1, this is how the stories we hold—sometimes expressed through triggers or implicit memories—start to speak through our bodies. In difficult boundary conversations, we may believe our safety or connection is at risk, and the imprinted belief from childhood comes back to visit: We begin to embody the idea that we can't set limits.

This was the case with Anya and Thanksgiving dinner. Her distressing feelings were resurfacing because this situation seemed so familiar to interactions she'd had with her mom as a child—even before she could speak. The unpleasant sensations associated with displeasing her mom triggered her mind and body to react similarly to the way she had as a kid—thus her fawn response and inclination to capitulate to her mom's demand.

At the core of the issue with Anya lies an important truth about boundaries: If we don't feel safe, we will struggle to set good limits. The way our bodies assess the safety of a situation or another person occurs through a phenomenon called *neuroception*, a term coined by Dr. Stephen Porges.[4] Essentially, it's the subconscious process our brain circuitry uses to constantly assess danger for us. When we consciously or unconsciously feel we aren't safe, our bodies automatically shift into hyper- or hypoarousal. This is an incredibly helpful instinct when we are in actual danger. However, the neuroception of folks who've grown up in physically or emotionally threatening situations can become skewed.[5] As a result, they are more quickly pushed out of their WOT. This sense is exacerbated if they feel they don't have a voice, choice, or way to set limits on experiences that feel threatening.

WHAT WE NEED TO FEEL SAFE

To be physically and emotionally well, we must experience safety in our bodies.[6] "Safety" in this context implies that we (1) are in our WOT; (2) don't feel threatened; and/or (3) believe we have the resources and support to keep ourselves safe should threats arise (for example, by setting limits).

What Safety Feels Like

Safety in our bodies feels solid, responsive, and aware.
Safety in our relationships feels like connection, vulnerability, and trust.
Safety with God feels like connection, belonging, and mystery.

———

Let these descriptions be starting points as you consider what safety looks like in your own life.

Doing the work required to set boundaries and feel safe as adults is critical if we are to learn to try softer. As we begin to change the implicit or explicit narratives we were given, honoring our limits and creating safety are vital. After all, how can we even begin to try softer with the most wounded parts of ourselves if we don't feel safe in the here and now? How can we develop the emotional bandwidth to connect and engage with other people in a healthier way?

Too often, though, it feels easier to decide that we don't really have a choice or that the cost of changing is simply too high. Certainly Anya wondered whether it would be easier to agree to host Thanksgiving than to stand up to her mom. Since the holidays are so emotionally charged anyway, Anya mused that maybe she should just wait until the new year to set limits. Yet Anya knew that if she overaccommodated her mom one more time, it might ruin their relationship, because the exhaustion and resentment were stealing all of Anya's peace.

I wonder if as you're reading this, you can almost feel that pull to white-knuckle it when it comes to meeting others' expectations. Wouldn't it be easier just to do one more thing, please one more person, finish one more project for someone—*Just one more thing, please!* The hustle, the people-pleasing, the disconnection from our bodies can feel so *normal*, can't they? Not only that, but the sensations of guilt or shame—like those Anya described—can feel terrible, which also serves to keep us from setting limits.

What do we really need in times like these?

We need the resources of an integrated brain and the embodied knowledge that we are beloved no matter what. As you'll recall, we have access to all these truths when we're in our WOT; we can connect to resources we already have, like safe relationships with others and God. And only then can we truly care for our bodies and honor who God made us to be.

The best part about all this is that God *wants* us to discover this peace. Science says so. Daniel Siegel points out that an integrated prefrontal cortex is able to secrete a substance called GABA that helps calm the amygdala—the fear center in our brains.[7] How beautiful is that?

TOP-DOWN COMFORT

I want to offer you three main tools as options to help you feel safe, remain grounded in the present, and pull from the wisdom you already carry. Together they facilitate top-down processing, which is deeply reminiscent of the way God calms us too.

Just as God is our good parent who comforts us, so He created parts of our brains (like the prefrontal cortex, which secretes GABA) that can soothe us.

Remember that in order for us to stay in our WOT, the prefrontal cortex needs to be online to help inhibit the lower parts of the brain. The cortex is then able to "connect" with and calm the amygdala, part of the emotional center of the brain whose main goal is ensuring our survival. The prefrontal cortex's response is similar to the way a parent is able to connect to and calm a frightened child. For example, in Colorado we often have big storms roll through with deep rumbles of thunder and dazzling lightning. Understandably, my young son, Jude, runs into my arms as soon as he hears a boom of thunder. Remaining calm and staying connected to Jude helps him understand that as long as we are in a safe place, lightning and thunder won't hurt him. (Of course, if we're in the middle of a pool when a thunderstorm passes by, I am the first to get my kids away from it.)

We can learn to do the same for ourselves. We can learn to recognize that some situations that make us feel unsafe are actually okay. At other times, it's appropriate to recognize that we need to leave a situation or set limits for our own safety. The work of learning how to tell if a perceived threat is real, and to know that it's okay to have a voice, is what trying softer is all about.

Learning to Assess Accurately

The first tool in accessing top-down processing will help us accurately evaluate a situation. Let's return to Anya's story. She truly didn't have many choices when she was growing up. One of the ways she began to set limits in adulthood was by using attentional control; in other words, by choosing what to pay attention to as a way to determine if she was safe in her present situation.[8] Many people who've experienced chronic little t trauma, like Anya, have a skewed perception of whether a situation is truly safe—their brains have difficulty telling whether the pain they're encountering

occurred in the past or is happening in the present.[9] Anya
wasn't experiencing a physical threat to her safety, but when
she began to consider standing up to her mom, she started
to feel as though she were still a ten-year-old kid who would
be berated for stepping outside her mom's expectations. In
a sense, attentional control helps her remember in present
time that though the experience was legitimately painful, it
happened in the past, and she does not have to allow herself
to be treated like that anymore.

In our sessions together, Anya and I practiced attentional
control by asking and answering the types of questions below:

> *If she did refuse to host Thanksgiving dinner, could her
> mom hurt her?* No, not truly.
> *Did she in any way need to abide by her family's norms
> now that she was an adult?* Nope, she truly could do
> what she thought was best.
> *If her mom distanced herself from their relationship as a
> result, would Anya be okay?* Yes. In fact, Anya wasn't
> sure she wanted a close relationship anyway.

Though this type of assessment won't necessarily be enough
to fully calm you in your own moments of anxiety, once you
can determine that you aren't in any actual danger, you can
move forward with other resources that can help quiet your
nervous system. You can also develop internal reminders to
connect yourself to the present, such as *I can leave whenever I
need to*; *I can set boundaries*; and *I can use my voice.*

Grounding

Another tool that has become invaluable to me and most of my clients is *grounding*, in which we use our five senses to keep us connected to the moment and ourselves. Grounding is one of the primary tools I use to bring myself and my clients back into our WOT. The basic idea is to nonjudgmentally pay attention to sensory information so that we can calm down our nervous systems, which allows us to move back into our WOT.

For example, when clients are becoming overwhelmed, I guide them through an exercise known as "I Am Aware."[10] First, I have the clients identify what they are aware of from a sensory standpoint. They typically say something like this: "I am aware of the temperature of the room. I am aware of the texture of the wall. I am aware of the firm ground beneath my feet. I am aware of a slight smell of citrus." They continue on until they feel connected to the present, which then brings relief from any disturbing emotions or sensations.

So how might someone use grounding while practicing boundary setting in real life? Let's consider Sarah's experience.

Learning We Have Choices

After three weeks in therapy, it was evident that Sarah was a bright, compassionate person, but she was also terrified of saying no.

"Sarah, just for something different," I said, "I want you to be in charge of how my chairs are arranged in the office today. I want you to notice, from a gut level, whether something feels comfortable to you or not. For example, do you like when I sit directly across from you, or would you prefer my chair slightly set off to one side?"

Sarah became deathly quiet.

"I mean, I don't know. You're the therapist; shouldn't you choose?" she finally said. "If I tell you how I want things, I'll feel like I'm doing something wrong, like you would think I was judging you or something."

I then asked, "Sarah, as you do a mental body scan, where do you notice sensations in your body?"

"Oh my goodness, I feel like they're everywhere. But especially I feel like my heart is racing and I'm out of breath. There's this weird pulling in my neck too," she said.

From this information, we were able to pinpoint that Sarah was getting outside her WOT, which made it difficult for her to believe that it was okay to tell me no.

Once we realized this, Sarah practiced attentional control to recognize she was safe in the here and now. Next, I encouraged Sarah to practice grounding. I asked her to identify what she was seeing, hearing, and smelling in my office. Once Sarah took a moment to ground herself, she realized that she really did have a choice in deciding how the chairs were situated during our session.

Sarah told me how she wanted our seats arranged that day, and in the future she told me any time her preference changed. Once she even pointed out that my chair was higher than hers and that she didn't like that. For us, on that particular day, this was a big win.

A few months later, Sarah told me that while she was out to dinner with an old friend, she had an opportunity to practice what she'd been learning. Sarah described how her friend was kind but at times seemed to steamroll over her opinion.

"After she told me for the third time that I didn't really know what was going on in our country, I could tell I was starting to get outside my WOT. Then I excused myself and went to the bathroom," Sarah told me. "When I was in there, I took a moment and reminded myself that Candace is my friend, but I am an adult and have the right to speak up for myself. I reasoned that the worst that could happen is she would disagree with me." This was how Sarah used attentional control to remind herself she was safe.

Next Sarah described how, while she stayed in the bathroom for an extra moment, she did a brief body scan and noticed she felt sensations in her neck and that her heart was racing. She wasn't completely flooded by her emotion but was nearing it. She then used our grounding exercise, taking extra time to put her hands under the water in the sink to feel the sensations on her skin.

"By the time I walked back to Candace, I still felt a bit afraid, but I felt like myself—not the little kid who couldn't say no. When Candace began pontificating on the same issue again, I told her I appreciated her opinion but didn't agree with it. I said I'd like to move on to something else."

Sarah had used her voice, remained connected to her body, and kindly but firmly communicated her boundaries. This, my friends, is what it looks like to try softer.

YOU'RE DOING BETTER THAN YOU THINK

I don't think it's an overstatement to acknowledge that setting boundaries is scary for many of us. Disappointing people *is* hard. And here's the thing: You will likely mess up as you practice setting limits. You will say yes when you mean no. You may take on too much at times. Perfection is not the point. It's about reestablishing your ability to honor your own voice, limits, and experience.

I've learned that setting boundaries is an essential element to my own emotional wellness—and there is quite literally no way for me to try softer without them. Yet at times I, too, fail to listen to my actual limits. And do you know what I need then? Compassion. I remember that it is courageous to use my voice and that honoring my experience is a sacred practice, because none of us graduate from our humanity.

I hope you feel empowered to recognize that even though you may not have had many choices when you were young, you have choices now. You can access resources to help ground yourself in the moment, keep your body calm, and, when you're ready, connect with your prefrontal cortex, which God gave you so that you can set healthy limits and do so with your head held high.

As you practice setting boundaries—and honoring your story, developing safe attachments, and becoming aware of your WOT—you will see the doorway out of survival mode. Dear one, we are invited to cease white-knuckling, because though it once kept us physically or emotionally safe, a new and gentler way is open to us. So now we come to the question we'll take up in the rest of the book: How can we begin trying softer right now?

TRY SOFTER

First, I invite you to make a practice of observing your here-and-now experiences to help build attentional control. For example, like Sarah, you could assess if a person or a room is actually safe and/or what choices you have. Doing this will help you access this information later if you begin to be triggered.

Depending on what is disorienting for you, you may also consider using these questions to help build attentional control:

1. Is my environment safe? (*The door is locked; I no longer live in my parents' household; the people I am with are trustworthy because* _____.)

2. What helps me remember I am an adult now? (*I have a job; I'm a parent; I graduated from college; I know how to solve problems when they arise.*)

3. What helps me remember I have choices? (*I could leave this restaurant; I could stop this conversation; I could ask for help.*)

Grounding Exercise

Before you begin, perform a body scan[11] and mentally notice if you feel connected to your body. You can do this by picturing a laser beam across your body that starts at your feet and moves up to the top of your head. Can you feel your breath? Do you notice any tingling or other sensations anywhere? Don't worry about figuring out where they came from; for now simply notice them.

Next, do the following to ground yourself in your present environment:

Name five things you can see.
Name four things you can touch and touch them.
Name three things you can hear.
Name two things you can smell.
Name one thing you can taste.

Now repeat the body scan. Do you notice anything different? Use this exercise when you begin to feel disconnected or overwhelmed to help you move back into your WOT.

Boundaries Script

If implementing boundaries is new for you or an area that feels tender, here are a few ways to help support you:

1. Notice your WOT. If you start to feel overwhelmed, return to the grounding exercise to give yourself a break.

2. First practice setting boundaries with someone you feel comfortable and safe with. That person might be your therapist, friend, or spouse. As you begin intentionally working on this

skill, notice what it's like when you name what feels good/best/preferable to you. Also observe how your limits are respected.

3. Create a script for yourself. For example, before ever saying yes to something, find a phrase that feels comfortable for you to buy yourself some time. Something like "Let me think on that" or "Let me look at my schedule" can be a good starter.

4. If you frequently find it difficult to set boundaries in a certain area, such as responding to difficult questions about family or making time commitments, create a script around that issue.

5. As you begin practicing boundaries, notice when your limits aren't honored. Allow yourself to take in this information and let it influence the strength of your boundaries with those people. For example, if you say no to people and they purposefully make you feel guilty or hold grudges, you might consider spending less time with them or communicating only when you have the emotional energy to do so. If someone continues to violate your boundaries, you might consider saying something like "I know it's disappointing when I can't do _____, but it really bothers me when you make comments like _____ afterward. Can you please stop?" Again, if someone doesn't adapt their behavior accordingly, this might be a sign that even stronger boundaries are needed.

PART 2

PRACTICES TO TRY SOFTER

WHEN WE HUNT

FOR BEAUTY,

WE LEARN TO PAY

ATTENTION.

CHAPTER 6

TRY SOFTER WITH YOUR ATTENTION

Listen, are you breathing just a little,
and calling it a life?

MARY OLIVER, "Have You Ever Tried to Enter the Long Black Branches"

FOLLOWING SEVERAL EXCRUCIATING YEARS of secondary infertility, Brendan and I were thrilled to discover I was pregnant. Up until then, we'd been told we had only a one percent chance of conceiving. I arrived at my seven-week ultrasound appointment as giddy as someone who'd won a major award, but by the time we left, I was overcome by hopelessness. The ultrasound tech tried to be gentle with the news, but the heartbreaking truth was that the baby wasn't developing.

All we could do was wait to see if a miracle would happen and the baby would begin growing again. So wait we did. First a week. Then two weeks. Our hopes were raised during the second ultrasound—the baby measured slightly bigger, and we were sure our prayers had been answered. Then in the third week, we learned our baby wasn't growing. And again at the next appointment—no more development. I felt as if I were slogging through mud during every moment of the twenty-four days we waited to see if our baby would someday breathe in my arms. Every day I cared for my then nearly four-year-old, trying to be present but fighting dissociation and fog. At long last we got our answer: Our baby would not live—not on this earth anyway.

Our hearts breaking, we scheduled D&C surgery. And it was then, the day before the procedure, that all the work I'd done to learn a new way to be in the world bloomed. I asked myself, *What is the gentlest thing I could do today? What is it that I need as I go through this torment? Tomorrow will be traumatic, but what might I do to prevent it from becoming unresolved trauma?*[1] I reached outside myself, too, for help—to friends, our church, and Jesus.

For the first time, in one of the most difficult, darkest experiences I've ever had, I allowed myself to try softer. That morning I left Matia with a babysitter and went to a movie— a funny one—by myself. And even though it was a comedy, I cried, but I also laughed. Next I walked aimlessly for a while. I listened to worship music. I prayed. I talked to my sister— she reminded me to be gentle. I went to bed early. I tried softer.

The next day, I had my first and only surgery and said good-bye to the baby who wouldn't be. It took weeks and months—a continual trying softer—but I found my way back to hope, which allowed the grief to unwind from my soul.

Reader, I can't help but wonder if you resonate with some part of my story. I can't help but think you, too, may be acquainted with grief and a life that never seems to work out. Perhaps you have lived in survival mode for so long, simply trying to get through each moment, that you have forgotten how to be present in one.

Learning to try softer won't automatically erase the pain of shame, anxiety, or trauma. It won't make people love you differently. It will not take away the wounds already inflicted. It won't give you a different childhood. But it just might change *how* you go through pain. And by now you know that the way in which you move through hardship matters greatly. It can predict whether something becomes integrated into your experience and loses its intensity or builds in power to the point that you feel it might overwhelm you.

If my miscarriage had happened even five years earlier, I believe I would have experienced it much differently. I suspect I would have tried to push through my pain, willing myself to look okay and not make a big deal out of our loss. I'm guessing I would have tried to ignore the fear and sadness welling up inside me until it came out sideways in fits of anxiety and attempts to numb what simply couldn't be ignored. Now I didn't pretend to have it all together, and I made a point to be kind to my body and my spirit. That's not to say I wasn't deeply sad; I was crushed. When our baby miscarried, I felt as if I had lost the dream of ever having another child.

Learning to honor my pain—to listen to my heart, mind, and soul—allowed me to respond with kindness and move toward healing.

And why do you and I need to learn this kindness? Because

if in our development we perceived that it was selfish to pay attention to our own experiences—maybe because we needed to be highly aware of our environments, maybe because we were shamed or were told we were bad—we might be unable to observe and attend to the rest of ourselves. We'll never truly heal.

Sometimes in my clinical practice, clients tell me heart-wrenching accounts of pain and abuse, but when I ask them to describe their emotions, they cannot do it—they simply cannot articulate how they feel. At other times, people have barely begun to share their stories when they dissolve in floods of tears or explode in outbursts of anger. They are what psychologist and author Kristin Neff calls "overidentified"[2] with their emotions. This tendency toward overidentification leaves them completely dysregulated—which is just another way of saying they were nearing the limits of (or already outside) their window of tolerance. Hear me when I say that neither tendency makes a person bad. They are natural reactions when we haven't learned healthy ways of tuning in to ourselves.

As different as their outward expressions are, what these clients share is an inability to pay compassionate attention to themselves—to not only observe their emotions but also consider how to be kind to themselves. Neff explains it this way: "Instead of just ignoring your pain with a 'stiff upper lip' mentality, you stop to tell yourself 'this is really difficult right now,' how can I comfort and care for myself in this moment?"[3]

For many of us, trying softer is exactly what we need.

MINDFULNESS: A CONNECTOR FOR THE BRAIN

As we've learned, a core part of trying softer is cultivating compassionate attention for ourselves. A great entry point for treating ourselves with kindness is mindfulness, which can be simply defined as "moment-by-moment awareness."[4] Like grounding, one of the reasons mindfulness is such a powerful tool is because research shows us that attention actually shapes our brains,[5] even in adulthood. In order for us to learn to try softer, compassionate attention is a primary tool we can use to rewire how our brains and bodies function.

The general practice of mindfulness is built on the concept of nonjudgmental attention. Many Christians use mindfulness with an intention to connect with God.[6] As Psalm 123:1-2 (MSG) says,

> I look to you, heaven-dwelling God,
>   look up to you for help.
> Like servants, alert to their master's commands,
>   like a maiden attending her lady,
> We're watching and waiting, holding our breath,
>   awaiting your word of mercy.

For centuries, Christian mystics and contemplatives have engaged in centering prayer, breath prayer, Scripture meditation, *lectio divina*, and other spiritual practices to help them pay attention to God's moment-by-moment presence, as well as to themselves. Jesus Himself invites us to live in the present by abiding in Him (see John 15:4). He tells us to notice the birds and flowers around us—reminders of God's ever-present care and concern for us—when our minds begin to fill with worries (see Matthew 6:26-28).

Mindfulness includes awareness of both external *and* internal things. This is one reason there is overlap in the meaning of contemplative Christian practices and secular/non-Christian practices. Practitioners of Westernized/secular mindfulness are simply looking to accept what is. But as Christians, we need not be afraid of this observing exercise, for we know that God holds it all: "Everything comes from him and exists by his power and is intended for his glory. All glory to him forever! Amen" (Romans 11:36, NLT).

The Catholic priest Richard Rohr explains it this way: "If you are present, you will eventually and always experience the Presence."[7] No matter how we come to understand presence and attention, it is evident that it is a helpful way for humans to exist in the world.

So how do we cultivate this responsive attention in our brains? As is true with so much higher-level thinking, we rely on the prefrontal cortex to be responsive rather than reactive with our attention; as we work to be mindful, the PFC will act as our internalized attuned parent to help us decipher what is helpful and what is not.

Recall how one function of the cortex is "to think about thinking."[8] In a sense, this is where we retain the ability to be mindful; we engage the top of our brains and use our attention to observe whatever we choose. For example, I may begin to mindfully notice that I am experiencing a sense of dread every time I consider making a particular phone call. If I am in my WOT and my PFC is online, I have the ability to observe this sensation in my body without becoming overwhelmed by what I'm experiencing.

Pema Chödrön uses this metaphor to describe the dynamic of mindfulness: "You are the sky. Everything else—it's just the weather."[9] Our ability to observe something without becoming "emotionally hijacked"[10] by the response of our amygdalas allows us to learn—even if slowly—to pay attention without getting overwhelmed by the intensity the experience brings up.

Through research, we've come to understand that when a part of the brain is utilized and strengthened, the gray matter in that part of the brain increases.[11] The more we engage in mindfulness, the easier it becomes and the more the gray matter is increased in the PFC and other areas of the brain.[12] This may be why, from a therapeutic standpoint, the generalized practice of mindfulness has significant mental health benefits, such as the following:

Practicing Mindfulness in Your Everyday Life

- Put your hands under the faucet and notice the temperature of the water. Wash your hands and notice the varying sensations.
- Go outside and put your bare feet on the grass. Notice the textures and shades, etc. Notice the leaves on the trees. Count them; notice their shapes and their colors.
- Hug a loved one for five seconds. Notice your breathing, your heart rate, and any accompanying emotions.
- Meditate on the verse "Your beauty and love chase after me every day of my life" (Psalm 23:6, MSG).

- reduced stress;
- lessening of chronic pain;
- improved emotional regulation;
- increased compassion; and
- heightened curiosity.

We were created to pay attention, a practice that helps keep our brains fully integrated. Learning how to be mindful of the sky, a tiny crack in the sidewalk, or the vibrant color of a flower can serve as a bridge to learning how to tune in to the frequency of our breath or the sensations throughout our entire bodies.

Last year I attended a training that incorporated mindfulness. Our instructor led us through an exercise to help us practice various types of awareness. First I noticed the entire room; then I focused attention on a beautiful magenta flower. Next, when the instructor asked me to hone in on one spot in my body, I noticed a specific place in my shoulder that felt neutral—with no pain—and finally I tried to hold a picture of my entire body in my mind and notice what was happening in all of these parts. For me, focusing on the flower and on one part of my body were the easiest.

The key to mindfulness is that we hold the things we observe with a posture of nonjudgmental awareness, simply noticing what is in our awareness rather than reacting to it. In my own experience, this is the hard part. But friends, this is a key step toward trying softer. It's difficult to build toward compassion—toward ourselves or others—if we continue to be highly critical of everything around us.

It's important to consider your WOT as you examine various practices, because just bringing your attention to your body may bring up unpleasant thoughts and emotions, so you may need to work up to that skill in the presence of a safe and skilled clinician. My husband has recently been trying to approach his life a bit more mindfully, and we've had many conversations about how hard it is not to immediately judge or try to fix what we are experiencing. For example, Brendan has found that practicing mindfulness requires more focus in the midst of a traffic jam than when he is drinking his favorite cup of artisan coffee at our kitchen table. It makes sense, doesn't it? In both instances, mindfulness is helpful, but one situation may require more practice than another. It's quite normal for people to find one form of awareness easier or more soothing; what's important is that we are paying attention.

Taking an observing approach is a good practice. Just like anything that our brain is learning to develop, it can take time to cultivate. Yet it is a skill that can be built, like a muscle. Stick with it.

BE STILL AND KNOW: THE POWER OF ATTENTION

Colleen experienced significant relational trauma as a child. Her mother died in a car accident when she was only six, and when her father remarried, her stepmother seemed to criticize her every action. While Colleen still felt close to her dad, over time it felt as though she were losing him, too, amid her stepmother's overbearing presence. During our work together, I explained the importance of learning to be attentive and compassionate to herself. At first she resisted, saying she felt she was already too self-involved (as her stepmother had constantly reminded her). Actually, Colleen had a small WOT, so situations moved rapidly from feeling tolerable to intolerable to her—and as a result, she sometimes experienced intense, unmanageable emotions that overwhelmed her, making her feel self-absorbed. That led to shame, and guess what happened next? She tried even harder to ignore and numb her feelings until they flooded through her again, and the cycle continued.

By now we know that our relationships with our caregivers, especially during childhood, dramatically affect the way we see others, God, and the world. If you learned it was selfish to pay attention to yourself, or if you have an insecure attachment style or have endured relational trauma, you are likely to have internalized the belief that your experience doesn't matter.

As a young woman, I sometimes heard messages in church that seemed to reinforce this idea, whether it was intended or not. When I was told that we should die to ourselves, I immediately decided I was selfish to try to make sense of my inner world. Yet I honestly couldn't imagine dying to myself any more than I already had.

I had always felt as if something were off inside me. Often after being with a crowd or in an emotionally intense setting, I would need long periods of time alone just to feel like myself again. I knew that was a clue to something important, but I was not yet able to put my finger on what it was. Meanwhile, the input I seemed to get from others was that I needed less of me. I was too much.

What I really needed was someone to help me be gentle—another important biblical idea—and to help coax the scared little girl inside me not to work so hard all the time. It wasn't until years later that my therapist (because, yes, therapists have therapists too) helped me understand how disconnected I'd been from my own internal experience, and for such a long time. As a coping skill, I had learned to tune in to my surroundings—so extensively that I'd lost touch with my own experiences and had tried to white-knuckle my way through life. This hypersensitivity exhausted my nervous system, often filling me with anxiety, dread, and neck pain. I came to hate this about myself and pushed myself even harder the next time—wondering if maybe I could just get over this part of myself and simply focus on others' expectations.

It wasn't that I needed less of me, I learned; it was that I needed to find a way to listen to the truest parts of me. While it might sound like a good and noble thing to be acutely aware of others but not of ourselves, it's not. When we are not paying attention to our inner worlds, we are susceptible to emotional burnout, exhaustion, emotional dysregulation, and chronic pain.[13] Because our brains are shaped around what we notice, it's important that we become better and more effective at listening—and responding—to what our minds and bodies are telling us. This is the journey of trying softer.

LEARNING TO LIVE WITH ATTENTION

What Colleen and I worked toward was this key under-standing: Simply being aware of an intense sensation is not the same as maintaining a mindful posture toward it. Picture the difference between being stuck outside in the middle of a rain-storm and watching a forecast of that upcoming storm while sitting safely inside your home. When you're in the storm—without an umbrella, no less—all you can do is react. But when you know the storm is coming, you can respond to the threat by staying inside or grabbing rain gear on your way out of the house. Instead of just reacting, you respond deliberately.

Bit by Bit: Pendulation

If you are just beginning to step into this mindful, present approach to life, it's important to know that it's okay if it feels challenging. As you learn to try softer through compassionate attention, you must also learn to pace yourself. Pendulation is one practice that will free you to do this, and it's something I coached Colleen to learn to do.

Even after she and I had worked together for a few years, Colleen's WOT was still fairly small. She had, however, learned to recognize if she was creeping out of her window by noticing when her stomach tightened and her body grew heavy, as though she were walking through mud. In our ses-sions, she showed great progress when she would interrupt me and ask to do some grounding exercises because it meant she was tuning in to herself. Sometimes she would get up and move around the room—simply trying to notice how she needed to respond in order to feel safe and connected.

Rejection was a major theme for Colleen throughout her day-to-day life. We could discuss it for a few minutes, but because of her painful attachment history, she had learned to disconnect from her body. As she went deeper into stories, I could see her fold into herself under the weight of the pain she still held; she called the feelings that came up "the black hole." "I'm trying to pay attention, but when I do, it makes me feel worse!" she would cry desperately.

As Colleen worked toward paying compassionate attention to herself, I introduced her to pendulation as a way of approaching these disturbing issues as they came up. In one of our sessions, Colleen chose to focus on a pink orchid, letting herself take in the texture and bright color. She noticed how it made her feel light and free.

From then on, when we began to process her deep losses, she could practice pendulating: first centering her attention on the pink orchid—something tangible that felt soothing or empowering—and then shifting her focus to something that might feel disturbing, such as feelings of rejection in her life now or the tightness in her chest as she thought of that rejection. As she did this difficult work, she would also "bring" the orchid resource with her, remembering that she could always shift her focus back to that if she became too overwhelmed.

By first spending time connecting to her orchid resource, Colleen was able to remain well inside her WOT as she briefly connected with the uncomfortable sensation. After a few minutes of swinging back and forth between the two targets, she said that the intensity in her chest had lessened.

Be gentle with yourself if, like Colleen, you find it challenging to learn how to extend compassionate attention to yourself, and see what it's like to pendulate between comfortable and uncomfortable sensations or emotions. You can't white-knuckle yourself into trying softer—but as you learn to gradually embrace even the hard parts of your story, the intensity of your pain will lessen, and you *will* move forward. Hold on to the truth as you are in the gray spaces of your life: You can and should find the goodness and glimmers of light along the way.

Beauty Hunting

Early in our relationship, my husband learned how much I adore sunsets. The way they invite us to notice the goodness immediately in front of us moves me. Growing up, I would sit on our deck in the evening observing the mighty Columbia River. My old hometown is situated on steep hills, and my parents' house was perched just right for a gorgeous view. As the sun set over the river, which was coursing its way into the Pacific Ocean, the sky's colors would gradually intensify and become golden.

As I write now, I almost weep at the memory of those beautiful sunsets. The colors would seep like watercolors across the sky, such vibrant reds, pinks, and oranges that I wished I could bottle them. The sunset would fade, and then dusk would outline the nearby mountain ranges in deep teals and intense greens. As time wore on, the stars would shine like diamonds. (I promise that one clear night on the coast could revive anyone's belief in God!) The way my family now notices the twilight is a bit of a running joke; apparently, I've stopped to point out a stunning sunset to them a few times. Brendan frequently asks our kids, "Did you know this is Mom's favorite time of night?" Everybody chuckles a bit, because they know. But even my seven-year-old will now stop and notice sunsets with reverence.

The truth is this: Long before I ever knew about mindfulness or emotional regulation, I knew about beauty. It has always been a way I've connected to God and a sense of myself. Just as the loveliness of an orchid provided rest for Colleen, beauty is an invitation and a resource to each of us.

When we hunt for beauty, we learn to pay attention. We keep our eyes open for goodness and for cracks of light. I adore how the late Irish poet John O'Donohue spoke of the complexity of beauty:

> Beauty isn't all about just nice loveliness. . . . Beauty is about more rounded, substantial becoming. So I think beauty, in that sense, is about an emerging fullness, a greater sense of grace and elegance, a deeper sense of depth, and also a kind of homecoming for the enriched memory of your unfolding life.[14]

The things that draw my attention and cause me to connect to this world are rarely manufactured perfection; instead, they are intricate and somewhat mysterious. This is why I offer beauty hunting as another resource for the work of cultivating compassionate attention. After all, the work of trying softer shouldn't feel like a bruising douse of pain from a fire hose. With beauty, it can feel like a homecoming.

Tracking

Another important resource I can offer you in your journey of compassionate attention is tracking, which is simply learning to intentionally notice your sensations and emotions as they change.[15] For example, if you notice there is pain in your neck during a tense meeting, or pressure in your chest after hearing about someone's grief, tracking may help you realize how you can find some relief when you move positions, change your posture, or attend to yourself in some other way. Tracking also allows you to respond purposefully to these sensations.

Several years ago, I began to realize that after a day of seeing clients, I would frequently come home with an intense muscle headache. This had been happening for years, but I would never really notice the pain until I was packing up and leaving for the day.

It wasn't until I trained under a wise trauma therapist that I began to understand that while seeing clients, I had not been tracking with my own experience for hours at a time. I would sit with folks and be deeply attuned to them, but in the process I would lose myself. Practically, this meant I had been ignoring or remaining unaware of the way I held my neck or my body and bypassing the cues of hunger and thirst that my body had been giving me. Over time, this pattern had taken a toll on me in ways that I couldn't quite articulate. I loved my job, but I couldn't believe how worn out I was all the time.

As I became curious about this dynamic, I realized I had been simply replaying a pattern I had learned as a child. Back then, my home life had been so chaotic that in order to endure the turmoil, I had to be tuned in to my external experience and ignore or dissociate from the sensations in my body. I had to pay attention—not in the mindful way we've been discussing but rather in a fear-induced, white-knuckled way. This—and I can't stress it enough—isn't the way you and I are meant to live. And the repercussions are real.

Somewhere along the way, many of us learned that to validate or pay attention to ourselves is wrong. If I had a nickel for every person who told me they think they are bad when they listen to their own body's experience, I'd be rich. To be clear, I'm not saying that what we experience is *more* important than what someone else experiences, but it is *as* important as another's experience. The apostle Paul encourages us "not to think of [ourselves] more highly than [we] ought" (Romans 12:3), but how ought we to think of ourselves? We know from Scripture that as Christ followers, we are image bearers of our God; we were known by our Creator in our mothers' wombs; we are temples of the Holy Spirit; we are members of a royal nation; and—my favorite—we are beloved. I think it's fair to say that as we honestly assess our own needs, we are absolutely thinking of ourselves as we "ought."

This is why I deeply appreciate the following words from psychologist and spiritual director David Benner:

Leaving the self out of Christian spirituality results in a spirituality that is not well grounded in experience. It is, therefore, not well grounded in reality. Focusing on God while failing to know ourselves deeply may produce an external form of piety, but it will always leave a gap between appearance and reality.[16]

Benner is articulating what many therapists have been saying for decades: Knowing about something is not the same as having an embodied knowledge of it. Curiosity and self-awareness matter a great deal in our journeys toward trying softer, precisely because they reveal what is at the deepest parts of ourselves.

LOVE YOUR NEIGHBOR *AS* YOURSELF

Attunement

Mindful attention toward our internal experiences is a step toward practicing self-compassion; in turn, it can lead to attunement—a responsiveness to our own needs. Attunement is built on attention, but it's not attention alone. Instead, it includes offering ourselves the same love and receptivity that God intended for parents to give to their children. Our heavenly Father is kind, responsive, and steady, and He made us with the ability to internalize the reality that we aren't alone and are worthy of love. Though some parts of our minds may believe God is good, the work of trying softer is treating ourselves in the same way we believe He already sees us so that we can more deeply experience the reality of how we are loved. Just as I want my kids to internalize my love for them, so God wants us to know our belovedness in the deepest parts of ourselves.

Learning to attune to ourselves is essentially the climax of trying softer—we are aiming to rewire our brains so they receive what they needed when they were young. It is the work of reparenting ourselves and participating with God's good design to help us heal and thrive by filling our toolboxes with practices that help us embody the truth that we are loved and valuable, even when those we are closest to can't be physically present. We are made for relationship—not just with others but also with ourselves. So attuning to our internal workings is the key that unlocks all the other parts of trying softer.

Because our brains are shaped around what we notice, self-attunement helps us become better and more effective at listening to the heartbeat of our own humanity. And here's what I truly love about the way we are designed: As we do our own internal work, we quite literally develop the capacity to listen to and love others more fully than before. Now it's worth saying that we don't do our work *only* so we will love others better—although it's a beautiful benefit. Nope, we are invited to connect to and respond to our internal world because we are deeply valuable and loved by God; and because that is true, we can rest in the fact that our needs matter.

Sometimes I feel a burst of joy as I consider how deeply interconnected people are and how our own healing allows us to help others heal too. The process of learning to attune to myself has taught me that the greatest gift I can give my clients, family, and friends is not my knowledge or even what I can do for them. Instead, when I'm connected to my embodied self, I can more deeply connect to them too. I've learned to allow compassionate attention to dance between us so that I can be with them and also with myself.

How is this possible? We know from neuroscience that as we feel our emotions, we have the capacity to feel *with* other people. This takes place in the conglomeration of circuits that Dr. Daniel Siegel calls "resonance circuits."[17] Essentially, a brain pathway called the *insula* connects what is happening in our bodies with the part of our brains that attunes to other people (using the mirror neurons we talked about in chapter 5). The insula then conveys this information to the prefrontal cortex, which brings it to our awareness. Have you ever sat with someone who was crying—and though you had no idea what was going on, you sensed that you might cry too? This is because your mirror neurons were tracking with that person's body, which then caused you to feel in your own body what was happening in theirs. When we are connected to our own internal experiences, we can "map" what is happening with other people too—even if no words are involved.

Jesus commanded each of us to "love your neighbor as yourself" (Matthew 19:19). In a quite literal way, the ramification of not living in tune with ourselves is that we are less able to connect to the experiences of others. (Of course, as we do this sacred work of loving others as we love ourselves, we must hold our own limits in tension, understanding that we are finite.) What beauty is available to us in this ability to connect with others.

Holding Space

Debra, one of my clients, looked me straight in the eye and said, "But you can't have gone through this before. This is too bad. Too ugly."

She was right. I hadn't gone through her exact hardship before, but I had been through other shattering things in my life; and more importantly, I was not afraid of her emotion— mostly because I had felt many big feelings in my own life. So part of my role was to bear witness to her pain in a way that felt safe for her.

We all need people who will spread their arms and create a space for us to be. We need them to see our lives and know us, whether we're being our messiest self or our best, most beautiful self. This essential need to be seen is part of how God put us together.

Doing our own work allows us to feel with others, and it is the framework that allows us to *hold space* for others. This is why therapists are (hopefully) required to go to therapy as part of their training. This is why it matters that leaders, parents, and pastors are aware of their own wounds and do *their own* emotional work.

While there is no absolute definition for what it means to hold space, I like to think about it as the process of carving out a sense of sacred space for people to experience what-ever they need to without shaming or rushing to fix them, remembering we are cotravelers on our journey through life.

As the body of Christ in particular, we are invited to

participate in this holy work of holding space. The apostle
Paul speaks to this idea when he says,

> Blessed be the God and Father of our Lord Jesus Christ,
> the Father of mercies and God of all comfort, who
> comforts us in all our affliction, *so that we may be able to*
> *comfort those who are in any affliction*, with the comfort
> with which we ourselves are comforted by God.
>
> 2 CORINTHIANS 1:3-4, EMPHASIS ADDED

Paradoxically, as we engage in our own deep emotional
work, we love each other in the most alive, empathic ways. We
do not see the people in front of us as tasks or obligations—
they are the *imago Dei*, and we see and feel with them.

For a long time, I struggled to believe that I, too, was
worthy of receiving this space in the same way I wanted to
give it. But I can remember feeling the crawl of slow change,
particularly when my husband and I were struggling with
another couple who'd gossiped about us, and I felt incredibly
misunderstood and alone.

I met a close friend of mine at the park, and while our
littles played, I honestly expressed my hurt and confusion. As
she received this, it felt as if someone had laid out a thousand
pillows for my soul to rest on. She didn't have advice for me.
She didn't judge me. She simply saw me. She honored my
sorrow. She validated what I was feeling in a gentle and loving way, and it made all the difference.

My dear reader, I pray you feel rich freedom to allow

yourself to listen—maybe for the first time—to the cries of your mind, body, heart, and soul. And then, as you're able, I pray you will make space for others to listen to themselves too. As St. Augustine prayed, "Grant, Lord, that I may know myself, that I may know thee."

Yes, may it be so.

TRY SOFTER

Pendulate with Beauty

1. First find something in your immediate surroundings that you notice is soothing, calming, or empowering.[18]

2. Spend a few moments observing it. What is its shape? Color? Texture? Smell? What do you enjoy about it? As you observe, allow yourself to sink into the soothing connection with this resource. Is there a name you could give the experience you are having as you connect with this pleasant object? Spend as much time with your resource as you want, and if you don't want to move into something uncomfortable, you can return to that challenging piece at another time.

3. Next, release the pleasant experience you've just had. Now begin to notice if there is an emotion or part of your body that feels uncomfortable. Remember, if at any time this experience feels overwhelming, you can stop and practice grounding (see page 111).

4. In your mind's eye, do a body scan (see page 111) and notice where you feel any other sensations or emotions.

5. As you identify the sensation or emotion from the last step, notice if it has a texture, a color, a size. Give yourself a moment to simply

notice it and stay with it briefly (for thirty seconds or less). Can you give a name to this sensation?

6. Now return to your resource. Allow yourself to breathe and fully focus on the comforting object. Notice yourself letting go of the uncomfortable emotion/sensation for now.

Interoception (Seeing Within)

1. Find a comfortable seated position. This exercise will take five to ten minutes. If for any reason you experience distress, please know you can discontinue the practice at any time. I encourage you to use grounding (page 111) to help you come back to a neutral place as needed.[19]

2. As you begin, soften your gaze or close your eyes, whichever feels more comfortable. Notice your breath. Don't try to control it; instead, just observe it. Is it shallow or deep?

3. Then bring your attention to your shoulder blades and your upper back. Notice if there are any sensations like heat or cold. Does this area feel prickly or sharp? Firm or soft? Using this same lens, observe your biceps, underarms, forearms, and hands. Simply notice what you're observing, knowing that God is with you in this space.

4. Next, allow your attention to travel to your neck, face, and head. Give yourself permission to move your neck or face gently, and continue breathing. Again, observe any sensations that come up.

5. Now bring your attention to your abdomen, lower back, and pelvic area, and down through your thighs and legs. You can move as quickly or as slowly as you feel comfortable. Continue down to your feet and toes, again simply observing the sensations.

6. If you're able, take a moment to stand up (if you're not able, you can do the same exercise while sitting). As you do, check in with the entire left side of your body. Now check in with the right side of your body. Does either side feel heavier than the other? Do you feel more aware of or more connected to one side of your body than the other?

7. As you're ready, come back to your breath and again observe its quality. You have just completed an exercise to examine the interior life of your body.

8. As a follow-up to gain better self-understanding, reflect on these questions:

   · What did you notice while doing this exercise?

   · Was it difficult?

   · Was there a part of your body that felt neutral or positive?

   · Are you sore? Hungry? Thirsty? Off balance?

   · Was there a part of your body that was hard to connect with?

   You now have more information about your own attunement to yourself. If, for example, you discovered that your stomach feels tight or uncomfortable, consider placing your hand on it as a way to support yourself. If you found that your shoulders are tight, consider allowing them to drop. If you notice that your arms wish to shake out some energy, give yourself permission to do so. In each of these examples, you are attuning to the need your body is presenting.

I PROMISE NOT TO

SEE MY BODY AS

SEPARATE FROM ME.

AS A COMMODITY.

AS SOMETHING THAT

MUST EARN APPROVAL.

JUST AS I AM THE BELOVED,

SO IS MY BODY.

CHAPTER 7

TRY SOFTER WITH YOUR BODY

Becoming the Beloved means letting the truth of our
Belovedness become enfleshed in everything we think,
say, or do.

HENRI NOUWEN, *Life of the Beloved*

I AM TWELVE YEARS OLD, standing in front of my smudged bedroom mirror in my green one-piece swimsuit. By anyone else's standards, my body is fine. But already I can see I am not the shape I should be. I do not have curves. I am square. Although I'm petite for my age, I pull at the skin around my stomach. *If only I had a waist*, I think. I'm already aware that a beautiful body—one that looks like those on magazine covers—earns attention and affirmation. And for now, having a beautiful body feels about as close to love as I can ever get.

So I want a different body.

I am twenty years old and a successful college basketball player who works out seven days a week. I am physically strong with tenacity buried deep in my bones. Even so, my body is not what it should be. I know this because I do not match the feminine picture of womanhood. I am not lean and lithe; I am muscular, with visible quadriceps from the hours of wall sits and defensive stances I've done during practice. I love my body, but I hate it too. All my working out—and the guilt, the shame, the restrictive eating—none of it is giving me the willowy look others prize. If only my clothes would fit my body the way I want them to.

I want a different body.

Now I'm in my midthirties. The concrete is hot under my feet as I hold the hand of my seventeen-month-old son and walk toward the splash pad at our community pool. We have just moved to the far-out suburbs of Denver, and I notice that most of the other moms here look so put together.

I feel a bit frumpy and quite self-conscious, if I'm honest. My skin is extrawhite, and my stomach feels fleshier than I'd prefer. A part of me wants to run and cover up. After all, I don't have the post–baby body I see all over the Internet. And a part of me grieves that we women walk around as though we need to constantly audition for an advertisement we didn't know we were trying out for.

I have believed I am beloved for so long. On this day at the pool, I realize that not every part of my body knows this and believes it—still. So I will try to live out my belovedness, even here. And I *am* grateful for this body that has carried so much; for what it has accomplished and for how it has held me, loved my children, and given me access to wisdom. I've mostly found peace with my body. I do not push it in the same ways I used to. Mostly, I try to listen to it now—to pour kindness all over those parts of me that have been plagued by my own criticisms and self-doubt. I am trying to live out what I already know—my body is me.

My tiniest and I finally reach the splash pad, and I settle into my breathing. Suddenly, a thought comes to me, a deal of sorts. I make a pledge to my body: I will not participate in objectifying my body or the bodies of those around me. I will not see myself as having to please other people through my looks, and I will not put other women in a place where they have to feel that way either.

I promise not to see my body as something separate from me. As a commodity. As something that must earn approval to be loved. Just as I am the beloved, so is my body. Just as my psyche deserves compassionate attention, so does my body. My body is me.[1]

So many of us were taught to fear, abhor, or disconnect from our bodies. As a result, we may mistreat or neglect them. Yet ultimately, we must learn to live in our bodies if we are to pursue wholeness and integrated lives in which we are connected to ourselves, others, and God. We must begin to listen to what our bodies are telling us about what has been done to them and what we are doing to ourselves. If we're going to try softer, we must continue our journeys of living in our bodies—being both gentle with and attentive to them. Why does this matter? Because learning to embrace our entire selves is not just a spiritual or mental endeavor—it is also an incarnational one. We must come home to ourselves.

Even now as I think about my own journey, I can recognize the shift from when I saw my body as something that existed to serve me to when I understood that it is the physical extension and expression of *me*. Viewing my body in this way is not just an idea; it must also be lived as an embodied practice. To do so, I've had to reexamine my thinking about my body and remember that it is so valuable and so loved that Jesus gave Himself for it:

> Don't you realize that your body is the temple of the Holy Spirit, who lives in you and was given to you by God? You do not belong to yourself, for God bought you with a high price. So you must honor God with your body.
> 1 CORINTHIANS 6:19-20, NLT

Since Scripture is so clear about the worth and workmanship of our bodies, why do we avoid the incarnational life?

FUNCTIONAL GNOSTICISM

In seminary, one of the classes from which I learned the most was church history. As I was taught about many of the challenges the early church faced, I realized that in some ways, their struggles weren't that much different from our own.

One of the primary heresies of the early church was Gnosticism. Essentially, Gnosticism teaches that anything spiritual—or having to do with the soul—is holy, and anything physical is bad. As a result, many attracted to this false teaching doubted the bodily incarnation and resurrection of Jesus. Though church leaders began to refute Gnosticism in the second century, we can still see its influence in the church even today.

In truth, many parts of Gnosticism don't integrate with the Christian faith—maybe its misunderstanding of why Jesus came to earth as a human being most of all. God's plan of salvation *required* Jesus to become fully human.

When Jesus entered the world as a baby, when He chose to become fully human while he was still fully God, He showed how much He valued our humanity and that He would do anything to save us—even if it meant death on a cross. He chose to vulnerably enter the world through the womb of a teenage girl and then to live with the risks, discomforts, and pain of being human. In doing so, He demonstrated that our personhood is not simply a tool and our bodies are not merely objects.

Jesus' body didn't just serve Him; it *was* Him. Jesus was His body. And, yes, He would later suffer, die, and be buried in His body before rising and finally becoming unconstrained by human limits again. But let's not pass over His thirty-three years on earth too quickly. Let's not rush past His death and sacrifice *in His body*, because His life on earth is a love letter to an aching humanity that teaches us how to try softer.

Jesus' life on earth says, *I choose to sacrifice My body so you can honor and pay compassionate attention to yours—this is the length to which I'll go to love you.* In the Gospel of Luke, He showed us the significance of His life and death at the Last Supper with His disciples: "Jesus took bread and gave thanks and broke it in pieces. He gave it to them, saying, 'This is My body which is given for you. Do this to remember Me'" (22:19, NLV).

Jesus came to show us the truest, best way to be human—not by denying His humanity but by embracing it. By living in it. By dying in it. And then, finally, by being resurrected in a glorified body. Jesus loves our humanity.

And Jesus' life on earth is why we can confidently say that God values our flesh and bones. He values the tears we cry and the hearts beating within each of us. He sees the emotional and physical bruises we've suffered. Jesus is tender to our humanity. He made it; He lived in its constraints; and He loves our bodies—just as He loves us. From Him we learn that there is no hierarchy, as the Gnostics said, to the physical and spiritual. It's all sacred, dear one.

The days I birthed my children were as precious as any prayers I've prayed, if not more so. The nights I sit by my children's beds, wiping their brows and tending to their needs—this work is sacred. Breaking bread with my husband, enjoying coffee with my friends, sitting with my clients in the midst of sorrow, stringing together words as I write another sentence, walking near the river and noticing the rhythm of the water and my breath—it all counts. There is no hierarchy. This is the embodied, try-softer life.

And when we are present to our bodies, we can listen to the needs they may be speaking to us. I have known many friends and clients who thought that if they could simply have enough faith or pray enough, their physical or mental issues would resolve. This is the spiritual equivalent of white-knuckling it. When we live an integrated life, we can sense whenever anyone—within our culture or the church—begins to value the spiritual over the physical.

Without realizing it, many of us still follow a sort of functional Gnosticism: We say God loves us, but we've internalized the belief that we have to punish our bodies because they don't reach a certain standard. We ignore, shame, or disregard our humanity. As a result, when we speak of God's love, we don't mean that He loves all parts of us; we mean that He loves our spirits. Or we pray as though we value our flesh and bones, but we don't think the pain we experience *in* our bodies affects our whole person.

We have internalized an implicit narrative that says the spiritual world is good and the physical world is bad.[2] This is significant on many levels, but through the lens of trauma-informed faith, we can see that the consequences are dire.

After all, for us as human beings, every issue we face affects the stories we hold in our bodies in some way.

We are not simply bodies walking around; we *are* our bodies. They are not all of who we are, but they are an essential part. We always pay a price when we try to live disembodied lives. The grief, anxiety, fear, or heartache we won't let ourselves feel will come out in other ways. As we discussed in chapter 2, each of our bodies is a system that longs for and is created to move toward healing. When we don't allow our bodies to process their experiences, they will certainly tell us—even if it means through panic attacks, chronic illness, depression, or more. Perhaps this is why the wildly popular and aptly named book *The Body Keeps the Score*, by Bessel van der Kolk, continues to resonate with so many folks. We know we can try to run from the wisdom and experiences of our bodies; after all, disconnection is one way we make it through uncomfortable relationships and experiences. But the truth is, our memories and experiences do not simply go away. Our bodies are their keepers, for better or worse.

LET'S PRAY AND GO TO THERAPY TOO

When I was a child, my parents began hosting prayer groups in our home during some of our most tumultuous times. The main purpose was to pray against and cast out any spirits that might be influencing the constant fighting between my parents or keeping any of us from experiencing

God's peace. The chairs in our living room were arranged in a circle so we would be ready for the Holy Spirit to move in our group that night. I felt a weightiness during those meetings—perhaps it was physical, or maybe it was spiritual. All I know is that I craved the nearness of people who might understand my family's pain, and I hung on to the tiny prick of hope that our dysfunction would be healed.

In many ways those nights of prayer were beautiful. Sometimes I thought, *Finally, we've believed with our whole hearts, and God is ready to heal us.* But the healing never came as I thought it would, and no one suggested there was any other way to restoration and peace.

Now, with the benefit of time, I can't help but consider that God might have worked to address our household's dysfunction through more concrete means, such as therapy or medication. While I was never told those things were wrong, there was always an undercurrent that if our belief was strong enough, God would simply heal us in an instant. What I've come to see is that just as God can heal cancer through modern medicine, He can use tools like counseling to rewire our brains. I know now that we were looking for an exclusively spiritual answer to a largely psychological and physiological problem.

Research now shows that trauma and emotional dysregulation literally change the way our bodies function.[3] As a child, I assumed that my chronic pain, severe anxiety, and sense of deep aloneness were signs that God was angry with me or even punishing me. I see now that I was simply

Ways Your Body Could Be Speaking to You

· Changes in temperature
· Sensations like tingling or heat
· Urges to move or flee
· Increase in heart rate
· Unexplained anxiety
· Unexplained heaviness
· Sudden alertness
· Feeling trapped or stuck

trying to hyperfunction as a member of a highly dysfunctional family. I was, in fact, a traumatized kid who needed not a longer checklist to follow but loving expressions of safety and care. I needed someone to try softer with me.

I believe Jesus intentionally interacted with flesh-and-blood bodies while on earth to show us a different way to live. I think of the man, blind from birth, whom Jesus and His disciples encountered in John 9. Seeing the man's need, Jesus spit on the ground and made a mud paste that he spread across the man's eyes. Then He told the man, "Go, wash in the pool of Siloam." The man did and then "came back seeing" (verse 7).

Did you notice that this man had to participate *with* Jesus in a physical way to be healed? This makes me think of how we participate *with* God as we pay compassionate attention to ourselves. What if when Jesus told the blind man to rinse off the paste, the man had turned to Jesus and said, "Thanks, but I think I'll wait till God heals me—you know, *the real way*." Oh my. I'm glad the blind man didn't do that.

Have you ever cut yourself off from a resource God wanted to use in your life? Have you ever completely discounted your physical experiences? I know I have, especially when I was younger. I thought, *Well, if I do such and such or if I listen to my intuition, will it mean that I don't believe God is big enough to heal me?*

Hogwash.

Listen: Jesus was certainly capable of healing the blind man on the spot. But He didn't. He took him through a *process*—a strikingly physical one.

WE ARE INVITED TO VALUE OUR BODIES TOO

How about you? Have you internalized the subconscious narrative that your body is worthless or bad? If so, you will be prone to objectifying, ignoring, numbing, or punishing yourself because, frankly, you won't think it matters.

Let's not fall for these lies. Our bodies matter. Our bodies are telling stories about our joy and our pain. And we are created to listen to their narratives. When we cut ourselves off from our bodies' sensations and act as if they didn't matter, the implications for our mental health are dire.

In the end, is it good simply to agree that our bodies matter? Well, yes and no. As with everything else we've learned about trying softer, we need more than just knowledge—we need an embodied experience of the truth.

To understand just how integrated our bodies are—in order to value our bodies the way that God does—we need to recognize that our brains are not just in our heads.[4] Quite literally, our brains are interwoven throughout our bodies. But how can this be? Researchers have discovered evidence for what many have known for a long time: The body is not just what transports the brain around; it is a highly interconnected system. And though important, the cortex is not the only part of the body that offers wisdom and insight.

Dr. Daniel Siegel discusses the complexity of the brain/mind/body in his book *Mindsight*. He writes, "By looking at the brain as an embodied system beyond its skull case, we can actually make sense of the intimate dance of the brain, the mind, and our relationships with one another."[5] As it turns out, our brains go beyond our skulls and into even our fingertips. Siegel also points out that from our earliest growth in the womb various clusters of neural cells begin creating what will become our spinal cords and brains. But some of those same neural cells become part of all the tissue in our bodies (like muscles, the heart, and skin).[6] In other words, the same neural cells that make up the brain also help form the rest of our bodies.

When we are aware of and attend to our bodies' sensations, we are practicing embodiment. According to Arielle Schwartz and Barb Maiberger, we rely on three sensory feedback systems within our bodies:[7]

Exteroception describes awareness of and interaction with sensory experiences outside our bodies. This includes sight, sound, touch, smell, and taste. Grounding and beauty hunting, two practices introduced earlier in the book, are examples of exteroception. When I go on a walk and smell the scent of freshly cut grass and notice the wind blowing across my cheek, my body is using exteroception to take in this information. These interactions with our bodies and the world around us help us feel supported, connected with others, and emotionally regulated, and they help us experience God in our world.

Proprioception refers to an awareness of the orientation of our bodies without having to consciously think about it. This especially takes into account how our bodies are positioned—whether lying, leaning, standing, or balanced. It is recognizing how our bodies take up space in the physical world. When I play games with my kids by hopping on one leg or throwing a ball, I am using proprioception to know what to do without having to consult my thinking brain on what my body should do.

Interoception relates to awareness of our internal states. Neurons throughout our bodies provide information to our brains about sensations such as hunger, thirst, pain, tension, body temperature, alertness, and thirst. As we go through the day and notice a heaviness in our chests, that our stomachs are growling, or even a sensation that we want to dance, we are experiencing interoception.

Though we didn't use the term, we first discussed interoception, which is a key part of trying softer, in the previous chapter.

Essentially what all this means is that our age-old understanding of mind over matter is flawed. There is no distinction between mind *and* matter; there is only us. You may
forget the technical terms for these ways of knowing, and
that's okay. What is important is that you remember to honor
and pay compassionate attention to your body.

———————

When I was about nine, I learned I could beat most of the
boys in basketball on the school playground. I started to
crave more time on the court, so one of my favorite things
to do was play pickup basketball at Peter Pan Park with my
older brother and sister, who were both talented in their own
right. Both of them were already in high school, so it was no
small thing to join them. When we were ready to go, I'd tie
up my pride and joy—my Charles Barkley Nike shoes—and
grab my well-worn ball. Something about holding a ball in
my hand and making a shot a girl wasn't supposed to be able
to make taught me that I had what it took to show up in the
world and to occupy space usually dominated by boys and
men.

I'm grateful for this experience, and when I feel insecure
or doubt myself, I often think back on those days as a
reminder of how strong and capable I really am. During my

college career, I wrote on my basketball shoes the Scripture verse my mom spoke over me when I was young: "Be strong and courageous. Do not be afraid; do not be discouraged, for the LORD your God will be with you wherever you go" (Joshua 1:9, NIV). The practice of remembering what it felt like to succeed strengthened me in those times when I was weary and scared. It's yet another example of what it means to pay compassionate attention to ourselves—to figure out what we need to be brave. This is particularly true for those of us who received implicit or explicit messages that it wasn't okay to take up literal space in the world.

As a counselor and a woman, I have seen how common it is, especially for females, to feel as if it isn't okay to honor our abilities, strength, and fire. My older sister and I discuss this topic often. During our phone calls, we take turns encouraging each other that it's okay to feel afraid when life seems difficult. But even so, somewhere in each of us is a strong, capable young woman who knows how to take up space on the basketball

Ways to Speak to Your Body

- Thank you for supporting me.
- You can take up as much space as you need.
- Thank you for the feedback you are giving me.
- I want to listen to what you have to tell me.
- You are worthy of good things.
- You can untangle the pain that is wound inside of you.
- I will keep you safe.

court and in the world. We take time to remind each other that we can trust that God created our bodies to be our allies and that they are giving us helpful information.

So how do we come to trust our bodies?

CULTIVATING A FELT SENSE

A core concept within embodiment is developing and beginning to listen to our *felt sense*. We experience this sense when we compile all the sensations our bodies are giving us to viscerally *know* something and create a larger picture of what's going on inside our whole selves.[8] Our felt sense adds to our ability to live embodied lives because it gives us feedback about how to be more deeply present to our physical bodies and attend to whatever they are telling us.

Have you ever walked into a room filled with friends and felt yourself shift into a state of warmth and excitement simply because you were there? Alternately, have you been with someone who had just received bad news, and without knowing what it was, you felt sad too? Both of these are examples of a felt sense. Listening to this information from our bodies helps inform what we do next. For example, in the first scenario above, I may find myself speaking with my hands and wearing a gleaming smile (both are expressions of embodiment that enable me to more fully experience the moment). In the second situation, if I notice heaviness and sadness inside me, I may attempt to connect with the hurting person by asking how they're doing, allowing my facial expression to mirror their sadness, or even asking if they'd like a hug. In a way, a felt sense helps inform how my body, brain, and spirit can remain aligned in these situations, and even how I can intuitively process difficulty. For our work of trying softer, a felt sense that is expressed through embodiment helps us to listen to, repair, and nurture the needs of our whole selves.

For all the reasons we've talked about—trauma, insecure attachment, shame, and more—many of us never developed the skills to listen to our felt sense. Or perhaps we have experienced this way of knowing something, but because we've learned to doubt and hate our bodies, we have ceased to listen to the information they give us.

Remember how in chapter 6 we talked about learning to love our neighbors *as* ourselves and how vital it is to be in touch with our own emotional experiences in order to connect with others? From a neurobiological perspective, we learn to be aware of our own internal physical selves through the insula.[9] It is considered the "superhighway"[10] that connects information from the body, lower brain, and mirror neurons to the middle prefrontal cortex. As with all of trying softer, the PFC is where we begin to make sense of what we're experiencing viscerally. This system is a vital part of our embodiment work.

Traditionally, intelligence has been thought of as a merely logical, linear way to understand the world. But our ability to remain open to the sensations and the felt sense of our bodies allows us to have a deeper intuitive understanding of ourselves, others, our environment, and even what the Spirit may be communicating. Rather than predicting how we will feel in the future, this information from our bodies gives us insight into how we're experiencing the world in the here and now. From this awareness, we have more tools and information to support us as we move forward.

For example, a few years ago I knew I needed to make some changes around how I managed my private practice. Through twinges of dread that would begin in my stomach and rise to my throat, my body had been letting me know that my current situation wasn't working. I realized I needed to build in more breaks, establish stronger boundaries, and end my days earlier. Though I considered that some people might think I was making these shifts for my own convenience, I sensed internally that I had to rearrange these practical aspects of my day-to-day life to honor my whole self. As soon as I listened to my body and took those small steps to give myself more breathing room, the apprehension began to dissipate, and I felt a renewed sense of hope.

Learning to love my body rather than just asking it to perform has certainly been a journey. It hasn't happened by accident, frankly. Trying softer in this way has been one of the most foundational aspects of my journey because my body is the home that holds me.

And how can we grow and change if we can't feel at peace in our homes? Physiologically, how can we process and learn if we don't feel safe with ourselves? This is an invitation for all of us. We are each invited to come home to our bodies in order to experience life in the truest way possible.

TRY SOFTER

When we live disembodied lives, we are not aware of the information our bodies are making available to us. One way we can begin to move toward embodied lives is by cultivating a listening posture around our felt sense. When I work with clients on body-based exercises, it's useful to reflect on these questions with them: *How do you know what you know? What is informing your experience? How can you say something is a "gut feeling"?* The following exercises will help you practice answering these questions and deepen your own felt sense.[11]

1. Find two or three pictures in magazines and lay them out before you. Choose one to begin with, and notice your initial reaction to it. Is it pleasant or unpleasant? How do you know? Notice in your body what sensations are coming up for you. Take a moment to observe them. Do you feel tense or soft? Engaged or disconnected? Do you feel light, heavy, jumpy, achy, or bubbly? What color would you assign to the sensation? Are you curious or repulsed? Simply give yourself permission to observe why you know what you know and where you are experiencing sensations in your body. As you feel able, do this with one or two additional pictures in the magazines and continue noticing all the sensations that are coming up at one time (all of these put together are your felt sense about that particular magazine picture).

2. Now collect several pictures of family or friends and do the same exercise. What are your initial reactions? Where do you feel each sensation in your body? Do you feel tense or soft? What color would you assign to the sensation? Are you curious or repulsed? Simply give yourself permission to observe why you know what you know. As always, keep your window of tolerance in mind as you engage this practice, and if your reactions become overwhelming, you can always shift your attention to something more pleasant with beauty hunting (page 128) or with grounding (page 111).

3. If you are practicing the felt sense exercise with pictures of family or friends and encounter a difficult sensation in your body, see if you can stay with the sensation for a few minutes. Consider placing a hand on the spot where you are feeling the sensation and—using the idea of tracking from chapter 6 (page 130)—observing if it changes.

   While staying with the sensation, you may notice the urge to cry or change your breathing, and all of this is helpful as long as you remain in your WOT. The changes you experience as you stay with your felt sense are signs that your body is processing what you are experiencing. Note, however, that simply bringing awareness to what you are experiencing is already part of trying softer, because you can't listen to, repair, and nurture what you don't know exists.

The understanding you gain from these experiences is your felt sense, and over time, it can help you integrate insights you receive from your body in an intentional way. For now, the main purpose of this exercise is to bring into awareness *how* your body knows something. You will need this information as you learn to try softer with your emotions.

It's important to remember that the definition of embodiment is noticing and attending to the sensations of your body, knowing that God made your flesh and bones and called them good. We can do just about anything in an embodied way; the critical piece is to bring our *attention* to it.

WHEN WE

APPROACH OUR

DISTRESSING EMOTIONS

WITH CURIOSITY

& COMPASSION,

WE CAN LEARN

TO SOAR.

CHAPTER 8

TRY SOFTER WITH YOUR EMOTIONS

Most of us were not taught how to recognize pain, name it, and be with it. . . .
But what we know now is that when we deny our emotion, it owns us. When
we own our emotion, we can rebuild and find our way through the pain.

BRENÉ BROWN, *Braving the Wilderness*

THE ROOM IS THICK WITH EMOTION as Kira shares her intense story
of pain and abandonment with me. As she talks, tears trickle
down her cheeks, slowly at first but then building into rivers.

The fan in my office whirs, and I wait, listening, doing
all I can to hear Kira and attune to her pain. As I sit across
from Kira, I breathe slowly, intent on creating the space she
needs to share. I sense the holy awe of this interaction as
Kira explains that no one in her family was allowed to talk
about feelings—ever. Whenever anyone did, or even tried,
they were met with shame and derision.

"We didn't do emotions," Kira whispers. "We didn't let
feelings stop us."

Near the end of Kira's seventh-grade year, her dad was

transferred to his company's headquarters on the other side of the country. Her mom quickly found a job there too. Kira was devastated at the thought of leaving the few friends she had finally made after an eternity of not fitting in. *How many years will it take to feel like I belong this time?* she wondered. After hours of pleading, she wore her parents down, and they allowed her to stay with some family friends so she could finish the school year. Her parents moved to their new home in early May, and a few days after classes got out, she would fly to her new home.

Kira had never flown before, so as the day of her flight approached, she was terrified. She thought her dad might empathize with her, but when Kira told her dad how scared she was, he laughed. "Don't be a baby! You've got it easy! Your mom and I had to drive in a hot rental truck for days. You'll get here in a couple of hours." As he spoke those words, Kira felt her hope buckle beneath the shame.

Her mom didn't empathize either. "Kira," she sighed when Kira hesitatingly asked if she could come back and fly with her, "you are just going to have to figure this out. I still have stacks of boxes to unpack, and I haven't earned any time off yet. You can't seriously be this scared?"

It was then Kira decided she'd do whatever it took to stuff down her feelings of fear and panic and make the flight. As she sat in her seat, terrified, the plane suddenly hit turbulence, and all she could think was, *If I go down today, will they even care?* That flight was just one of many times when Kira's parents minimized or ignored her feelings. In response, Kira learned to white-knuckle it through every hard thing—until she couldn't anymore.

For years, Kira stuffed her feelings with anything she could: food, relationships, exercise. Later, she tells me, she felt detached from her emotions, and she turned to alcohol as her drug of choice to remain disconnected anytime they surfaced. It was easier than feeling them. But once she tried to quit drinking, she found herself overwhelmed by her emotions.

Because she hasn't dealt with her feelings for so long, it takes Kira several sessions to identify the root issues she wants to address. As she processes her pain and empties her heart, she tells me she feels emotionally exhausted but also deeply ashamed.

"I have a husband who loves me and beautiful kids who adore me—and still, I can't get away from this grief. I know people have it worse than me. I know I should be thankful," she says. "One minute I'm terribly angry at myself for being so selfish, and the next I feel stuck again—lost in a wave of emotion. I hate myself. I hate that I'm so weak. These things happened thirty years ago! I want to forgive. I have forgiven, but my heart—it's shattered still. Why does it still bother me?"

In every sense, I'm aching as Kira shares her pain. At the same time, I'm not surprised by her contempt for her emotional experience or her sorrow. I've heard such self-condemnation many times before in my own life and my clients' lives.

SHAMING EMOTIONS

After several years in Christian counseling and extensive training in trauma and emotional regulation—and to be honest, just living as a human in the world—I became aware of a trend: People *love* to criticize emotions. Whether our own or others', emotions are often used as a scapegoat for what is wrong with just about anything.

Do any of the following statements sound familiar?

Don't listen to your feelings—they'll always lead you astray.
Your feelings are sinful.
You shouldn't feel that way.
Having feelings makes you weak.

One of the ways we keep ourselves from paying compassionate attention is by disconnecting from our emotions or shaming ourselves when they won't be ignored. As a person who loves Jesus, this made me wonder, *How do I reconcile the idea that I am a deeply emotional and sensitive person with the common narrative that it's not okay to honor our feelings?*

Are difficult emotions sinful? Do we simply need to silence our feelings? And if that's not the answer, what is?

DAVID, A MAN WHO FELT ALL THE FEELINGS

It doesn't take much biblical study to see that God created us as emotional beings. When I think about deep feelers, I can't

help but think about King David. This was a man who loved
Yahweh and was also a profound sinner. Yet this complicated
person is also known as "a man after [God's] own heart"
(Acts 13:22, NIV).

As the author of many psalms, David frequently spoke to
God with intensity:

> My heart is trembling inside my chest
> as the terror of death seizes me.
> Fear and dread overwhelm me. I shudder before
> the horror I face.
> I say to myself, "If only I could fly away from all of this!
> If only I could run away to the place of rest and peace."
>
> PSALM 55:4-6, TPT

> I spread out my hands to you;
> I thirst for you like a parched land.
> Answer me quickly, LORD;
> my spirit fails.
> Do not hide your face from me
> or I will be like those who go down to the pit.
> Let the morning bring me word of your unfailing love,
> for I have put my trust in you.
>
> PSALM 143:6-8, NIV

Does King David sound like a person who's trying to
pretend or to stuff his feelings? To be clear, I'm not suggest-
ing that we all need to feel our emotions *exactly* like David

did, but I suspect God knew what He was doing when He allowed us to read these big expressions of emotion.

Another heartening reminder of the value of our emotions comes from Jesus' interactions with his friends Mary and Martha after their brother, Lazarus, died. The shortest verse in the Bible sums up Jesus' response to the people grieving near Lazarus's tomb. It simply says, "Jesus wept" (John 11:35).

Jesus absolutely knew what was about to happen. He knew that even though his friend had died, He would be raising him back to life momentarily, but—and don't miss this—Jesus *still* wept. What kind of God is this? He honored and entered into the present grief of His friends. They had just lost their dear brother—*of course* they wept. Jesus didn't shame them; instead, He validated their humanity.

When Jesus lamented with His friends, He was allowing them to process their emotions. As He joined them in grief, He had to know that experiencing their feelings was allowing them to tap into their bodies' natural ability to integrate difficult experiences. As the Creator of their neurobiological structures, I suspect He even recognized that their limbic systems needed to move through the emotions they were feeling so the pain didn't become a form of trauma. Notice that this God-in-flesh did not rush Mary and Martha along but instead provided empathy and patience. This is a model for us as we seek to pay compassionate attention to our own experiences.

This might sound strange to most folks, but Jesus' weeping

is one of my favorite things to talk about. This is the Jesus I know and serve and give my life to; the One who holds the redemption story in one hand and the fragility of our human emotion in the other—and loves them both.

EMOTIONS GIVE LIFE

Through examples like David and Jesus, we can see that embodied, alive people have—and embrace—emotions. To try softer, we need the information that emotions give us so we can know how to respond to ourselves. As Peter Scazzero says in *Emotionally Healthy Spirituality*,

> To feel is to be human. To minimize or deny what we feel is a distortion of what it means to be image bearers of our personal God. To the degree that we are unable to express our emotions, we remain impaired in our ability to love God, others, and ourselves well.[1]

Researchers are still seeking to understand all the elements that enable our bodies to generate emotions. Much of the way we name and even experience emotions is contextual and cultural.[2] For example, Jesus would have known and experienced grief for His friend Lazarus in the specific setting of His Jewish culture and family. So even while emotions are universal, the nuances by which they are expressed may vary. Each of us learns or constructs emotions based on

elements like our environments, histories, and caregivers—
and this fits the science around attachment. In a sense,
emotional response is one way our bodies express the stories they hold. Understanding this helps us to recognize
why there is a clinical distinction between our emotions
and our feelings:

> The *sensations and nervous system states* that we
>   experience in our bodies = Emotions
> The *names* we give those expressions = Feelings[3]

Let's further unpack the distinction between our emotions and feelings. As we've already explored, our bodies
play a much more significant role than most of us realize as
we learn to try softer and stay in our window of tolerance.
Yet when we've learned to white-knuckle our way through
life, emotions and feelings can seem as if they are happening to us; as a result, we don't recognize that they are first
evoked in our body. If I had known as a college student
that the stomachaches and constant neck pain I experienced
were connected to my emotions and unprocessed trauma,
I would have better understood what was going on in my
body. I simply assumed that my feelings were experienced
only in my brain, completely separate from my body. Now
we understand that before we know something is happening in our conscious mind (including our emotions), we
know it first in our body. Once we've brought our bodily
experience and sensations into our conscious mind, we can

name what is happening and thus have the ability to do something with it.

So whether or not you use the terms *emotions* and *feelings* interchangeably (I still sometimes do), what I want you to see is that in order to feel our emotions in a healthy way, we must continue our integration with our bodies. We must recognize that when we cut ourselves off from our bodies, we cut ourselves off from our emotions too. In order for us to try softer, we must recognize that healthy emotional awareness always includes the body.

For a moment, will you consider what life would be like without an emotional experience? What does a symphony sound like when we don't have the resonance in our bodies? What does a day out with our kids look like when we don't pause to recognize the beauty and experience gratitude? What does a broken heart mean if it does not cause pain? How do we learn that our words or actions are hurtful if we receive no reaction? What does love feel like with no emotional connection? Why should a baby continue to giggle if we don't crack a smile in return?

Emotions add texture to our lives. They are the feedback to our interactions. They are a response to our stories, physiology, and environments—those parts of our lives that make us who we are. They are the balance to the cerebral brain, and we need the information they give us. When we don't learn to name and become familiar with our emotional experiences, we don't have a vocabulary for what we're experiencing, which can leave us feeling disoriented and cause parts of our brains to be disconnected from one another.[4]

LIST OF FEELINGS

Nearly fifty years ago, psychologist Paul Ekman identified six emotions he said are shared by people in every culture. The list below starts with those basic emotions and then provides many more gradations. Though it is certainly not complete (and some feelings may cross categories), referring to this list may help you identify your feeling. Why is that important? Research shows that naming your emotion may calm your limbic system and support the integration of your brain.[5]

Happy	Sad	Angry	Fearful	Surprised	Disgusted
Amused	Blue	Aggravated	Afraid	Astonished	Cynical
Carefree	Burdened	Agitated	Alarmed	Confused	Disillusioned
Cheerful	Depressed	Bitter	Antsy	Curious	Disturbed
Excited	Despondent	Brooding	Anxious	Delighted	Embarrassed
Exhilarated	Disappointed	Cranky	Brooding	Enchanted	Exasperated
Giddy	Discouraged	Cross	Cautious	Horrified	Fed Up
Grateful	Drained	Defensive	Despairing	Impressed	Humiliated
Joyful	Gloomy	Frustrated	Frightened	Incredulous	Jaded
Loved	Grief-Stricken	Furious	Helpless	Inquisitive	Jealous
Merry	Hopeless	Hostile	Hesitant	Intrigued	Offended
Optimistic	Lonely	Impatient	Insecure	Mystified	Outraged
Relaxed	Melancholic	Rebellious	Nervous	Puzzled	Repulsed
Satisfied	Pensive	Resentful	Rattled	Shocked	Revolted
Thrilled	Remorseful	Scorned	Stressed	Skeptical	Scandalized
Tranquil	Troubled	Testy	Tense	Startled	Sickened
Upbeat	Weary	Upset	Worried	Wary	Smug

If there's so much evidence as to why we need and should even *want* emotions, why do so many of us try to cut ourselves off from them?

Before I became a therapist, I might have been more willing to say we should just tell our feelings to knock it off. And that was once my normal response—as a trauma survivor, I have empathy for why we choose not to feel. I can remember that when I tried to prepare for tests in high school, I'd become easily frustrated with sadness or fear that would surface, believing they were only distractions. I'd tell myself, *Stop it! You are being bad. This isn't a convenient time for you to feel sad/mad/frustrated/anxious. You have work to do.*

I can see now that because I'd learned my emotions were a liability, I didn't think my feelings were worth listening to. Had I known my body was giving me signals that I was worn out and weary, I might have viewed my experiences differently. My body wasn't trying to keep me from success; it was telling me my emotions needed compassionate attention and that I was afraid I would be worthless if I failed.

Now certainly there are times when we need to healthfully contain an emotion, only to come back to it later so that it might be attended to and processed. Some days when I meet with clients, I am tired after getting to bed late or discouraged after an argument with my husband. It's important, however, that I don't use my clients' time to feel *my* feelings. (If your therapist does that, please find a new one!) I can't always process all the emotions that come up during everyday situations either. Though my impulse might be to yell at the person who cuts in front of my kids and me in the line at the grocery store, I am better off internally acknowledging my frustration and later asking myself why it brought up such fury inside me. Frankly, part of living is recognizing that we don't always have the capacity to work through everything that comes up at all times. However, this is different from living our lives as though emotions don't exist or don't matter. Even taking a moment to name what we are experiencing has been shown to integrate the right and left hemispheres in our brains and to calm down the firing in our limbic system.[6] Dr. Daniel Siegel calls this phenomenon "name it to tame it."[7]

When we've been socialized to believe that our emotions are weak or not allowed, we never create the neural circuitry to better regulate ourselves. How can we know how to be kind to ourselves or gentle to what we're feeling if we deny those emotions exist?

EMOTIONS HELP US

Imagine you wake one morning feeling fairly calm. You are walking to the kitchen to grab coffee when, with alarm, you notice your back door is cracked open. It appears someone has broken into your house. Suddenly your heart begins to race, and you experience fear, urgency, and panic. This reflects a shift from an integrated neurological system to a disintegrated state. Physiologically, this means that blood flow has stopped to certain parts of your brain, and it is no longer fully connected within itself.

If a friend calls you right then and tells you, "Oh, it's fine—stop being scared," will that take away the panic? Or the fear? Or the worry? Of course not!

So why in more everyday situations do we take the same approach with other emotions—our sadness or grief or anger—and expect that strategy to work?

We are physiologically unable to just *stop* feeling.

Instead, the way back to integration, or a whole brain, is to honor the signals our emotions are giving us, allowing us the ability to respond appropriately. Sometimes when we are afraid, we may need to call 911; at other times, we may need to allow ourselves to recall that the threat has passed and we're safe now. If we are with friends, they can reassure us that we are not alone and that experiencing powerful feelings is normal. In any event, it's vital that we attend to what is happening in ourselves.

This is important not only when we have an emergency but also when we receive a difficult email or hear painful news from a friend. As we've discussed, even when we can't fully process an emotion in the moment, it is important for us to notice what we're feeling[8] and give ourselves permission to name and honor what's there, knowing we can come back to it later. Taking these steps actually defuses the intensity of our emotions. Because we haven't repressed the sensations, they actually have less power. Once we consciously identify what's going on, we have more choice as to how and when to attend to it. The more frequently we do this, the better our entire selves become at trying softer.

LIFE IN THE EXTREMES

The truth is, even if we do choose to deny our emotions, they don't actually disappear. Just as with everything else on our journey through life, our bodies remember. If we ignore, numb, or disconnect from our emotions, the wisdom of our bodies *will* find another way to communicate to us. As Romans 8:22 expresses, all creation is groaning and longs to move toward healing.

Those of us who've had difficulty living from a place of emotional health typically have one of two experiences: Either we feel cut off from our emotions or we feel overwhelmed by them. As you'll recall, this is tied to our WOT and our physiological ability to tolerate our experiences:

Overwhelm (e.g., when emotions feel big or too much) = hyperarousal

Disconnect (e.g., when we are unaware of or not connected to emotion) = hypoarousal

Some folks oscillate between the two extremes without ever finding a comfortable middle place (WOT) with their emotions. This was the case for Kira, whom we met at the beginning of the chapter. At times she was overcome by her emotions, and at other times she found unhealthy ways to detach from them. Neither of these options allowed her to truly process her experiences or live fully present and engaged with her life.

So what does this mean for you and me? How do we

identify if we are either disconnected or overwhelmed by our emotions? The lists below may provide some clues.

Signs of emotional overwhelm include the following:
- Experiencing a sudden loss of what you actually think or believe (e.g., at a family get-together, a cousin tells you he was admitted to an Ivy League law school and you suddenly find yourself believing you've never been capable, when all along you've succeeded academically)
- A sense that you *are* your emotions, rather than *having* emotions (e.g., after your boss gives you some uncomfortable feedback, you find yourself unable to focus on anything but the sense of disappointment and self-contempt—even though she also complimented you on several areas)
- Inability to calm down
- A sense of being "swallowed up" by emotion
- "Knowing" the right answer but being unable to believe it
- Feeling physically wound up

Emotional overwhelm may present as anxiety, anger, or rigidity.

Signs of emotional disconnect include the following:
- Inability to identify emotions or sensations
- An experience of underwhelm in perceivably emotional situations (e.g., you tell a heart-wrenching story with no facial expressions or feelings)

- Knowledge of how you "should" feel, with an inability to connect with those feelings (e.g., after you give birth to a beautiful baby, everyone keeps asking if you are happy, but you realize you are not feeling much at all)
- A notable lack of desire or energy
- Feeling physically heavy or suddenly exhausted

Emotional disconnect may present as depression, lack of motivation, or appearing unaware.

Both overwhelm and disconnect, in a sense, make us less ourselves. Yet the answer isn't to vilify our emotions or our humanity. Instead, we must learn to move through our emotions—to tolerate them but also learn to take breaks when needed. As we do this, we create the conditions that allow our bodies to metabolize our experiences. When this happens, our bodies process our emotions and experiences in such a way that they stop feeling intense or disturbing and become moments, ideas, or memories that we can reflect on and assimilate into what we've learned.

When I describe this process to clients, I explain this work as being like putting a file in its correct location. Emotions, experiences, and sensations that are fully processed are filed in a part of our brains that our whole selves have access to, while emotions that never move fully through our systems (often because of big T or little t trauma) don't have the same access to our whole brains and continue to feel disturbing or intense.

LEARNING TO TOLERATE EMOTION

I sometimes think about our tolerance for emotions and/or sensations as a muscle we can strengthen. Take Kira and her fear of flying. Because she was never encouraged to *name* her experience and never felt it was okay to ask for support, she essentially buried the signals her body was giving her. She learned to ignore the shaking and the anxiety and tried to employ a "mind over matter" approach. In the absence of a caregiver who could help her understand it was okay to have emotions, her tolerance for emotions shrank. Her muscle was weak.

Similar to the way the muscles in our bodies atrophy when we don't move, so our capacity to sense and live into our emotions diminishes when we ignore them. We must open ourselves to an awareness of our feelings so that we can learn to tolerate them (and as always keep our WOT in mind).[9]

After many sessions with me, Kira decided it was finally time to deal with her intense fear of flying. By her own admission, she had spent years plagued with

How to Process an Emotion

1. Begin by observing your body in your mind's eye.
2. If you are feeling any sensations, determine where you are experiencing them in your body.
3. If it feels supportive, place your hand on the part of your body where you feel the sensation.
4. Take a moment to breathe and simply notice the sensation without judging or trying to fix it.
5. Notice the sensation that is connected to an emotion.
6. Observe how the emotional intensity peaks like a wave and then begins to dissipate.
7. If you can, name the emotion or experience you are having without fixing or judging it. If needed, refer back to the "List of Feelings" on page 172.

———

Note: If at any time you feel like you are going out of your WOT, you can choose to begin grounding or another containment exercise.

179

devastating anxiety attacks any time she needed to travel. In one sense, she reported feeling "totally fine" about flying and lacked compassion for herself around why she would feel any other way. But whenever we discussed an upcoming flight for a business trip or vacation, her body would begin to shake, and without any reason she could name, Kira would start crying. Over time, Kira and I worked to connect with the compassionate witness in herself (prefrontal cortex), name her emotional experience as it was happening, and recognize that there are no wrong feelings. As she went further in her work, she found more resilience. We also used the therapeutic approach known as eye movement desensitization and reprocessing (EMDR)[10] to help her address her fear of flying and several experiences from her childhood (including the cross-country move when she was twelve) that had added to her anxiety.

And yet none of this work with Kira would have been possible had she not been able to embrace, and thereby tolerate, the idea that her emotional self is part of what makes her human; it's part of what makes her whole.

We, too, can strengthen our emotional muscles by incorporating these principles for better emotional health:

1. **Name the experience.** As we discussed above, taking a moment to simply note our feelings can have profoundly positive effects. Researcher Lisa Feldman Barrett coined the term *emotional granularity*, which is the ability to identify and articulate the words that

AUNDI KOLBER

most closely match our experiences. She notes that the more closely we identify our experiences, the more it seems to help us regulate.[11] For example, my two-year-old recently stood in the middle of our living room and, while stomping his feet, yelled, "I'm sad, Momma!" I couldn't help but notice that he actually seemed quite angry at the moment—most likely because I'd told him he couldn't have a Popsicle until after dinner. Though I'm no perfect parent, I reflected back to him, "I see you're having big feelings. You can be sad, but I wonder if you're also mad?"

"Yes, I mad!" he yelled back as his little chest pushed out with intensity. Though his emotions didn't immediately dissipate, he let me hug him, and then we moved on to something else. That moment confirmed for me that feeling truly understood speaks to our deepest needs as humans. This is what emotional granularity does for each of us; it's like pinpointing a place on a map that we need to find. Whether we do it for ourselves or someone else helps us articulate our feelings, naming them is helpful. Additionally, strategies like tracking (introduced in chapter 6) help us better understand how our sensations and the way we experience them are changing. Remember, there are no right or wrong feelings; they just are.

2. **Ride the wave.** Not long ago, a dear friend came over with her kids for a playdate. It had been a while since

I'd seen her. As we talked about all the big and small changes in her life, she looked me straight in the eyes and said, "Remember all those years ago when you told me about riding the wave of emotion? It's one of the best things I've ever learned."

We both exhaled and laughed, because yep, we know.

Emotions, I had told her, are like waves, meaning the experience of an emotion forms, builds toward its peak, and then decreases. Often if we can tolerate staying with the emotion for thirty seconds to a minute, we find that it will peak and then dissipate.

When we recognize that emotions give us information and that it is normal for them to change, adapt, and even disappear, we can approach them differently.[12] This idea can be particularly helpful for folks struggling with anxiety, but it applies to all emotions.

3. **Practice containment.** If they haven't been processed, traumatic experiences can be reactivated when we are triggered, which can lead to intense emotion and sensation. In fact, the original experiences were traumatic in part because our nervous systems and bodies felt overwhelmed by them and didn't process them fully.

As we're learning to emotionally regulate, it's important to recognize that when something feels too big, it's not only appropriate but vital to use resources like grounding or containment (see pages 111 and 87).

While I am a big advocate for learning to feel our emotions, we must always keep an eye on our WOT so that experiences don't become retraumatizing.

As you practice containment, your goal is to have a felt sense that the distress has lessened, and though it may need to be processed at a different time, it no longer has the same immediacy.[13] One of my clients imagined a fire as the container in which she placed her distress. After watching it burn, she imagined herself picking up the ashes and spreading them from an airplane. At the end of her visualization, I sensed a visceral calm within her.

4. **Employ curiosity.** In addition to staying with our feelings, learning to soothe ourselves, and taking breaks when we need them, adopting an internal posture of curiosity is also fruitful. Curiosity helps brains that may be acting from the subcortical regions, such as the limbic system and amygdala, to reconnect to the cortex. When this happens, we acknowledge that the emotion we are experiencing is not the ultimate truth; instead, we recognize that it has information to share with us. From this higher level of thinking, we can then lovingly say to ourselves, *Hmm . . . that's interesting. I wonder why I had such a big reaction to making a mistake*, or *I'm curious why my heart started beating faster when so-and-so started talking about a family trip*. This approach allows us to get as much

information as possible so we can compassionately work through our distress.

5. **Speak grounding statements.** The final piece around emotional regulation is learning to recognize that we have feelings but we are not our feelings. From this place we can use grounding statements such as the following:

I am safe.
I can make choices.
I am capable.
I am lovable.
I am valuable.
I am in process.
I can set boundaries.

You might want to add to this list any other affirmations that help you move through emotion.

LIVE AWAKE

Many people assume that to be fully human means that we should be happy all the time. Life here on earth, of course, doesn't allow for that; instead, it elicits both pleasant and uncomfortable emotions. People who are aware of and know how to attend to their feelings are truly awake. They have learned to be compassionate with themselves even in difficult experiences so they aren't overwhelmed or cut off from their emotions. And the best part is, others can feel that same sense of equilibrium in themselves, too, simply by being around them. This is the sweet fruit of trying softer.

As you give yourself permission to have emotional experiences, some emotions may feel too big to handle on your own, and it's okay (and wise) to seek out support and help. Sometimes we simply need to give ourselves permission to take in just a bit at a time and then take a break—this is also completely normal, especially for folks who've lived through chronic trauma.

But most of all, I hope you understand that you are not weak for having feelings. You are not "less than" because you react to the world around you. Your grief, joy, anger, disgust, or fear does not define you, but it is a clue to what's going on inside you—and this is where the beauty happens. As we honor our experiences, we gain more freedom to move through our emotions rather than become stuck in them. Like Kira—who was so terrified by the thought of flying that it made her shake—when we approach our distressing emotions with curiosity and compassion, we can learn to soar.

TRY SOFTER

Emotional health occurs when we are neither overwhelmed by nor disconnected from our feelings. The following exercises are designed to help you get back to a place of equilibrium when you find yourself in either extreme.

Addressing an Overwhelmed Rhythm

(for those who overidentify with emotions)

Remember that it's vital to remain in your WOT as you move through emotion. If you sense you are nearing the edge of your window, use grounding or containment to ensure you stay within it.

1. In a journal or in another place to write, give yourself permission to name any emotional experience you are having. It may even mean naming a mixture of emotions. (To help you get started, use the list of feeling words on page 172.) Resist the temptation to judge the feelings you are having; instead, just name them.

2. As you observe your experience, scan your body and notice if you feel any sensations accompanying the feelings. For example, if you are anxious, where do you notice that in your body? If you are happy, where does that show itself? If you are experiencing a distressing emotion and it would be comforting to do so, place a hand on the part of your body that is experiencing the sensation. Notice the pressure and observe what that feels like.

3. As you are comfortable, invite God to meet you in whatever emotional experience you are having. Is there wisdom that can help inform your emotions? For example, if someone close to you hurts you and you're feeling frustrated, can you name your feeling but, as a way to help you stay regulated, also draw from past experience that this person is typically well-intentioned?

Addressing a Disconnect

(for those who feel disconnected from their emotions)

If at times you experience no or very minimal emotional responses in situations where it would be appropriate, consider trying these practices:

1. Begin by doing a body scan, and notice if you feel connected to your body. If not, take three short, shallow breaths from your chest.[14] As you do, simply notice the sensations in your body. While you are considering a situation that has some emotional charge and observing the sensations in yourself, ask,

   · Does this sensation have a shape?

   · A size?

   · A color?

   · If this sensation could talk, what would it say?

2. Now, refer to the list of words (feelings) that describe emotion on page 172. As you do so, consider what emotions might connect to the sensations you are experiencing in your body. Is there more than one word that might connect to your experience?

NO MATTER
HOW HARD WE TRY,
WE CAN'T HATE
OR SHAME OURSELVES
INTO CHANGE.

CHAPTER 9

TRY SOFTER WITH YOUR INTERNAL CRITIC

Be excessively gentle with yourself.

JOHN O'DONOHUE, *To Bless the Space between Us*

I HAVE LONG ADORED the idea of kindness and compassion. While in high school, I would lie on the floor of our old house and take in a worship song that put a tune to Psalm 145:

> The Lord is gracious and compassionate,
>   slow to anger and rich in love.

> The Lord is good to all;
>   he has compassion on all he has made.
>
> VERSES 8-9, NIV

As I sang along, I believed these words with as much of myself as I could. But I couldn't live as if they were true. I wanted to move with the freedom that comes from knowing I could receive the kindness God offers. I wanted to let myself believe that God's posture toward me was gentle, gracious, and compassionate. But I couldn't fully receive this truth because my internal critic was too strong.

Every time I failed to meet my own rigid expectations, the words I spoke to myself were far from loving: *How could you have been such an idiot? You should have seen that coming. You are too much. It's all your fault. No one wants you around anyway.* Whether I'd done something to set my dad off or missed a key shot in a basketball game, my first response was often to blast myself for not doing more or being better at life. I punished myself for being human—internalizing and sometimes even magnifying the judgment I felt from others. I tried ignoring my sadness and exhaustion, and I stayed on high alert in an attempt to avoid making another misstep. I wanted to live from the conviction that God's love was good—but that desire wasn't enough to overcome my self-hatred.

THE PIT OF SHAME

Have you ever felt this way? Have you ever been trapped in a cycle of frustration, anger, or criticism directed at yourself?

In my work with clients, I find that self-hatred/contempt is the most pervasive reason folks continue trying to white-knuckle their way through life. To be clear, there is nothing wrong with identifying our weaknesses and attempting to improve in those areas. There is, however, a big difference between healthy guilt and shame:

Guilt = I did something bad.
Shame = I am bad.[1]

From a faith perspective, we can think of healthy conviction as a motivating factor that leads us to repent of, or change, our actions. This is a beautiful, necessary part of growth and learning to try softer. Ideally, our caregivers model this for us when they repair relational ruptures. We all need a healthy sense of personal responsibility to help us love others well. For instance, I may immediately regret snapping at my daughter for laughing too loudly and waking her baby brother napping in the next room. As I see a flush of hurt spread over her face, I may scoop her into my arms and apologize, wishing I could take back my words and simultaneously offering myself grace by recognizing that, like many busy moms, I sometimes react without thinking. This is healthy guilt.

Healthy guilt allows us to recognize that we are loved and valuable even though we are imperfect. When parents prioritize love and safety in their interactions with their children, kids internalize a sense of connection, empathy, and personal responsibility toward others, and their nervous systems remain regulated. They can then receive feedback and gentle correction regarding their behavior.[2] This is why a secure relationship with God can be such a resource to us too. Even if our attachment styles do not allow us to be tender with ourselves quite yet, we can still experience God as a safe landing place. We can connect with Him, knowing He provides the security we need to work on our faults without despair.

Shame, on the other hand, is a critical assessment that *who we are* is not valuable, lovable, or worthy, and therefore we are undeserving of connection—and it is often rooted in the way our caregivers interacted with us. Developmental shame frequently "accompanies childhood trauma."[3] In fact, because of the way shame affects our nervous systems, we can actually call it little t trauma if it isn't followed by repair. In my experience, the primary difference between guilt and shame is this: The first recognizes that in order to truly change behaviors (or anything else), we need love, support, and regulated nervous systems. Shame, however, leverages the threat of relational exile as a way to teach (e.g., "Stop complaining or don't show your face around here"). One of the many problems with shame is that any change it stimulates in us will be only temporary. This is because it leads us to react out of our lower brains, where survival is the only goal. Authentic growth will always include our whole, integrated selves.

As I think about shame, I often think of this quote from author Peggy O'Mara: "The way we talk to our children becomes their inner voice." In a sense, much of our inner critic is fueled by unresolved areas of shame from our childhood. Just like other disturbances that affect our functioning, shame can have serious consequences. Those of us who grew up with significant internalized or toxic shame likely have a narrow window of tolerance, which we know causes us to react quickly and extensively, without our fully integrated brains, to even the smallest obstacles.

This, my friends, is precisely why we are choosing to try differently. Many of us have an internal voice that is keeping us stuck, traumatized, unhappy, and alone. This voice reminds us that we are not enough, not worthy, too much, and too little all at the same time. It's not hard to see how this voice impacts our day-to-day lives, is it? If our central narrative is that *we are bad*, then nothing we do will ever be enough—and no amount of behavioral management will fix this wound. Many of my clients have tons of information about "how to" live differently; in fact, information is never the problem. For instance, after we have discussed ways they could strengthen their relationships, they may start difficult conversations with their spouses, risk rejection by reaching out to new neighbors, or pledge to listen patiently to their surly teens. If their attempts do not go well, however, they often blame themselves for not being enough and castigate themselves for even attempting to connect better with others.

Trying softer isn't about *knowing* or *doing* the right thing; it's about being gentle with ourselves in the face of pain that is keeping us stuck. Because no matter how hard we try, we can't hate or shame ourselves into change. Only love can move us toward true growth. This is the love given

Try Softer Affirmations

- I have choices.
- I can set boundaries.
- It's okay to disappoint people.
- I am capable.
- I am loved no matter what.
- I am valuable.
- I can ask for support.
- It's okay to need help.
- My emotions give me information.
- My body supports me.
- My body gives me information.
- I am responsible for only myself.
- It's okay to take care of myself.
- This emotion is temporary.
- I am beloved.

to us by a gentle, kind, compassionate, good God—and the love we are invited to give ourselves too. Kristin Neff, the foremost researcher in the field of self-compassion, points out that compassion is different from empathy in that empathy is feeling with someone else, whereas compassion means to suffer with someone and then allow ourselves to be moved by that pain so we are motivated into action.[4] Our ability to be compassionate with ourselves strengrhens the internalized secure base within us and therefore calms our nervous systems, giving ourselves the attachment repair that we may not have received as children.

As I have walked through my own story, I have found the concept of self-compassion to be a transformative part of healing. Frankly, compassion is transformative not only for those of us who've have childhood trauma of some kind but also for all of us who were parented or taught to think that toxic shame produces growth. It's for each of us who has been stuck in the rut of self-hate. It's for every person praying for growth but finding it never happens. This compassion is the ingredient that allows us to truly access the love and acceptance we already know are ours—to integrate, open up, and create new neural pathways between our wounded parts and the loving, gentle ones.

UNDOING SELF-HATE

As a therapist, I have watched how keenly my clients' internal critic affects their well-being. Take Courtney. She was in her late twenties, dressed in the trendiest clothes and appearing quite confident when she first arrived in my waiting room. During our first session, I was curious about what areas of her life she wanted to work on, because she seemed self-aware, kind, and fairly calm. After we had discussed her childhood and several interesting stories from her travels, we neared the end of the session. Then I asked, "What would you say your main goal is for our work together, Courtney?"

Suddenly, Courtney's demeanor transformed, and the confidence I had seen melted away. "I—I keep sabotaging dates with perfectly good guys I'm interested in—I guess."

"Can you tell me more?" I asked slowly.

"Well, most recently there was a man that I've been friends with for a while. I asked him out to coffee, and it went great. He texted me the next day, and even though I'd had a fabulous time, I had this running commentary in my head that he was way too good for me, and what's the point of even trying? I ended up ignoring his texts because I figured it was just easier—he'd probably dump me anyway. Ugh. I've read at least thirty books on dating and stuff and it never helps! The advice never helps! I always come back to the same place—my inner critic tells me I'm worthless."

The reality is, many of us were raised to believe that we should be our worst critic and that being hard on ourselves was the best—maybe the only—catalyst for change. I often ask clients with a critical internal voice whether they would ever talk to someone else that way—or would ever allow another person to talk to them like that. Of course, the answer is generally no. Even more important, this condemning spirit contradicts the approach of our gracious, compassionate, and loving God. What if this intense dislike of ourselves is keeping us from embracing the truest thing about each of us—our belovedness?

How then can we begin to offer this compassion to ourselves? Neff identifies three main elements: mindfulness, self-kindness, and common humanity.[5]

1. **Mindfulness vs. overidentification.** Earlier in the book we discussed the practice of mindfulness and the way it helps us cultivate attention and strengthen the prefrontal cortex. Another benefit of mindfulness is that it gives us the ability to observe something in a

nonjudgmental way, allowing us to honor our suffering without getting stuck in the emotion.

According to Neff, pairing self-compassion with mindfulness is key to our ability to respond gently to ourselves. If mindfulness is about noticing our experience, self-compassion is about doing something with what we now know without becoming overidentified with the experience. For instance, during therapy Courtney learned to observe how her body would become activated anytime she thought about going on a date. She worked to simply notice that her neck would tighten, and she felt a sense of pressure in her chest that made her feel out of breath and hopeless. Once she could nonjudgmentally track her experience, Courtney began practicing compassion toward herself, using exercises she learned in therapy. Over time, she built up the tolerance to act in alignment with her true self rather than from a place of reaction and fear. Courtney's self-compassion made her resilient.

As with any practice of mindfulness, we aim to remain in our WOT as we do this, so that if we start to become overidentified or overwhelmed with an emotion, we can use a grounding skill and come back to the emotion later. However, once we can tolerate observing an emotion, the other pieces of self-compassion can be quite powerful.

2. **Self-kindness vs. self-judgment.** When we practice self-compassion, we extend the same kindness to ourselves that we might lend to a stranger, a friend, or a loved one. Instead of thinking we deserve harsher treatment than others, we give ourselves grace.

Often when working with people who have difficulty being kind to themselves, I ask them to think about someone toward whom they feel a sense of love or compassion, which makes it easier to direct those same feelings toward themselves. From a faith perspective, we know God feels tremendous compassion toward us. What if we let ourselves experience that compassion too?

When I recently asked a client to do this, she told me about her five-year-old niece, whom she adored. Then I said, "I know you're struggling to give yourself gentleness right now. I wonder if you could picture your niece alone and sad."

"Yes," she slowly replied.

"Okay, I want you to give yourself a hug, like you might give your niece a hug if someone told her she was worthless. Can you do that?"

She sighed. "Yes, I'll try."

I was grateful she was willing to do so, because the truth is that physical touch—even from ourselves—can release oxytocin in our brains. This is the hormone/neurotransmitter that allows mothers and babies to bond with one another, that's released when we fall in love, and that helps us feel more loving toward ourselves too.[6]

At the end of the chapter, we'll explore more tangible ideas on how to extend kindness to ourselves.

3. **Common humanity vs. isolation.** Suffering is not isolated; it's common to all humanity. Our world is broken. Sin exists. We are fragile. When we recognize that we are not unique in experiencing suffering, we are more likely to see ourselves as worthy of compassion. We are also less likely to feel as if we are alone; instead, we feel more connected with the human experience.

When we think of friends in our lives who are also struggling, we remember that though the sources of their pain are different, we are not alone, and this can make a huge difference to us.

This three-pronged approach is extremely helpful in our work of trying softer, in part because it enables us to learn to tolerate our feelings without getting stuck in them.

A KIND, GOOD GOD

If you're anything like me, you might be starting to wonder, *So is this actually what God wants for us—to love who we are unconditionally?* It seems too good to be true, doesn't it? After all, how will we change or grow if we're not shaming and criticizing ourselves? How will we stay in line?

It may help to recognize that God has *always* extended such kindness, compassion, and goodness to us. The Hebrew word *checed* appears often in Scripture and, according to Strong's Lexicon,[7] is most commonly translated as *mercy, kindness, loving-kindness,* and *goodness.* In the Old Testament, the term *checed* is used 248 times to describe this facet of God, as well as the way people relate to one another.[8] Obviously, we can see this is not a fleeting aspect of God's character but something He consistently displays.

The term that seems to be most difficult for translators to convey is the idea of loving-kindness. Some translators break down its meaning in such a way as to say it is *love that acts.* God's love combines generosity *with* responsiveness.[9]

In Psalm 25:6, the English Standard Version uses the term "steadfast love" for *checed*:

> Remember your mercy, O LORD, and
>   your steadfast love,
>   for they have been from of old.

The Amplified Bible, on the other hand, uses wording similar to that in the King James Version:

> Remember, O LORD, Your [tender] compassion
>   and Your lovingkindnesses,
>   For they have been from of old.

Language struggles to convey the depth of goodness that is present in God's character—the way we are wrapped in His love and the way kindness has always been a part of who He is. Pause here and really consider this with me—the kindness God extends to us is exactly as lovely as we dare to think. We don't have to keep living from a narrative of self-hate when God looks at us tenderly, waiting for us to move toward His fiercely gentle love.

Something that has always struck me about the idea of compassion, especially for Christians, is that we are constantly invited into an upside-down way of living. This is the foundation of who Jesus has always been—the God who says that the way up is down; that the way to become first is to be last; that you become strong in your weakness and face hatred with love—even, and maybe especially, if the one you hate is yourself.[10]

Reader, I want to invite you to see yourself as one who is gloriously loved and deserving of kindness and compassion. Every person struggles in some measure with the internal voice that tells them they are not who God calls them to be. And yet again and again He lovingly meets us and reminds us that we are the very ones He came for.

Perhaps this will be your faith walk throughout your lifetime—to gently step toward the truth of who you are in Him.

WITH LOVE TO THE YOUNGER ME

I stand on the edge of the deck at the back of my parents' former home almost ten years after they sold the house—a move that symbolized the breakup of our family. It's surreal to be here.

The house, which was built in 1901, is an eclectic mixture of Victorian and Craftsman styles with a touch of Japanese influence. The new owners have made a few major changes to the house since I've been here last, but the house's bones are the same. After I explain that I had lived here for almost twenty-four years, the family living here now kindly allows my husband, daughter, and me to look around. I feel the odd sensation of both grief and hope as I walk through the home. The wood floor still shines, but the kitchen has been renovated, and my long-standing mental picture of my mom working at the sink feels shaken. It's odd to hold the past and present together in one space, but I do; and I feel God's nearness with me as I take it in.

After touring the house, I return to the deck. I smell the salty air and gaze out at the view that grounded and encouraged me through so many difficult years. My breath still catches as I take in the 180-degree view of the mighty Columbia River. The day is overcast, which is expected in this small Oregon coast town. Even in late May, no one here feels entitled to sunshine. We'll have to wait a few more months for any promise of actual heat.

I turn my attention back to the home where I felt so much pain and joy, and I feel I am doing—at least symbolically—what Samuel did after God delivered the Israelites from their enemies the Philistines: He erected a large stone as a memorial and called it Ebenezer ("stone of help") (see 1 Samuel 7:7-12). Likewise, I mentally raise my stone of remembrance in gratitude for the victories God has won thus far. Returning to my childhood house now feels momentous and symbolic because I finally feel whole, loved, and valuable. Not perfect, certainly—actually, I feel less perfect than ever. What feels startlingly different from my younger years is primarily the deep sense of compassion I have for my younger self.

Looking back toward the river, I breathe deep and notice an ache in my heart as I remember her: desperate to be okay, longing to be loved, fighting to be known, and rarely experiencing peace in her soul. This is the moment I place my hand on my chest and whisper to my younger self, "I know you are scared. I know you felt so alone. You are not alone anymore. I will help you. We are more loved by God than we could possibly imagine."

I look over and see Brendan. And I know, deep in my heart, that all this is true. I have come a long way, and I am beloved.

TRY SOFTER

Practice 1: Speak Compassionately to Yourself

This exercise and the one that follows have been adapted from Kristin Neff's work. This first one will allow you to walk through the three elements of self-compassion in an area that is causing you distress.[11]

1. Place your hand on your heart, allow yourself to inhale and exhale, and simply notice what this feels like.

2. Next say these words to yourself:

   · *I am experiencing pain.* (Observe your emotion mindfully without judging it.)

   · *I am not alone.* (Remember that we are all surrounded by many others who have suffered or who are suffering.)

   · *May I be gentle with myself.* (God is deeply kind and compassionate with us, so we can be the same way with ourselves too.)

Practice 2: Connect to Yourself through Another

If you are in a situation in which you feel emotionally stuck and are struggling to be compassionate toward yourself, the following can be a helpful exercise:

1. First, picture someone in your life with whom you feel a connection and have empathy for. (This person could be a close friend,

spouse, or child, or even a mental/actual picture of your younger self.) Allow yourself to notice where you sense these feelings of connection in your body. Notice the quality of your breath and any other sensations that arise.

2. Now allow yourself to picture this person struggling with the same issue you are. What would you say to them? What advice would you give?

For example, a while ago I completely forgot it was my daughter's school-spirit dress-up day. As I dropped her off at school, I saw other students decked out in school colors and realized my oversight. I immediately felt a pit forming in my stomach and tightness building in my chest. I began to struggle with thoughts about what a terrible mom I was and feeling that I was not really there for my kids.

But as I realized what was happening, I pictured a dear friend of mine making this same mistake. Once I did, I began to feel lighter in my body. I saw myself comforting my friend. I realized that if she had struggled with this, I would have told her she's doing a great job in spite of that slipup. I was then able to turn toward the shame I was feeling and realize that, as always, it wasn't telling me the full story.

Interestingly, while my daughter had been a little disappointed when we pulled up to the school that morning, by the end of the day she had completely forgotten about it. When I apologized again after picking her up, she even told me, "It's okay, Mom. Everyone makes mistakes."

3. As you try this same practice for yourself, consider placing your hand on your stomach or chest as a means of recognizing and empathizing with your internal discomfort.

Practice 3: Practice Loving-Kindness Meditation

Many people use a loving-kindness meditation like this one as a means to mindfully approach themselves and the world in a more compassionate way. Because I believe God is the One who loved us first and who makes it possible for us to love Him, ourselves, and others as we should, I have adapted this practice to reflect a Christian perspective. Please feel free to adapt this exercise further to best meet your needs.

1. Sit comfortably, either in a chair or on the floor. Notice your breathing and focus your attention on your heart. Visualize your breathing coming in and out of this area. Try picturing a beam of calming light shining directly into this area of your body.

2. Now recite the following to yourself as you breathe from your heart's center:

   May I experience Christ's love.
   May I experience Christ's peace.
   May I experience Christ's presence.
   May I experience Christ's compassion.

3. Now think of someone toward whom it is easy to direct feelings of loving-kindness. Recite those words again, this time inserting the person's name:

   May _____ experience Christ's love.
   May _____ experience Christ's peace.

May _____ experience Christ's presence.
May _____ experience Christ's compassion.

4. Finally, as you feel comfortable, extend this blessing to all the earth and its inhabitants:

May all creation experience Christ's love.
May all creation experience Christ's peace.
May all creation experience Christ's presence.
May all creation experience Christ's compassion.

THE HARD THINGS
THAT CRACKED US OPEN
HAVE THE POTENTIAL TO
CREATE SPACE FOR DEEPER
JOY & RESILIENCE.

CHAPTER 10

TRY SOFTER WITH RESILIENCE

I have come that they may have life,
and have it to the full.

JOHN 10:10, NIV

ONE COLD AND SNOWY DECEMBER NIGHT, I woke up knowing this was the day. Nearly thirty-eight weeks pregnant—and just eleven months after my devastating miscarriage—I knew I had gone into labor.

Glancing at my phone in our pitch-black bedroom, I saw that it was only 3:00 a.m. As I contemplated waking my husband, I remembered that he had a 6:30 a.m. business meeting and let him sleep. Minutes later, contractions began working their way through my body. As I reached over to wake him, he grumbled, "But, honey, I can't reschedule this business meeting."

Slightly annoyed, I touched his shoulder one more time, "Hey, hon, I know it'll be hard, but I'm having a baby today, sooo . . . you're going to have to."

That got him going.

Brendan shot right up, and bless him, he started apologizing and gathering our stuff. Once Matia's babysitter arrived at 5:30, we headed to the hospital. Traffic was nearly at a standstill as drivers navigated through one of Denver's only major snowstorms that winter. I breathed slow and deep, praying silently that the drive wouldn't take as long as it looked it might.

Brendan looked at me and said, "We got this, honey. We'll get there." He said it so confidently that I instantly felt calmer.

After we settled in at the hospital, my contractions seemed to slow significantly. I gave my body time to do the work it was naturally created to do, walking the halls and having a lighthearted conversation with Brendan and the nurses. Then, just before noon, something changed—dramatically.

As the pain coursed through my body, I thought to myself, *Keep going. Breathe.*

In that moment I knew one thing: Keeping our bodies relaxed sounds good in theory, but when it comes time to practice it, it's much more complicated. I had created a birth plan, with the goal of laboring on my own as long as possible and then asking for pain medication when needed. Once the intensity of my contractions increased exponentially—going from a pain level of 3 to 10 in just a few minutes—I asked for an epidural. As I shook with the waves of the contractions, time seemed to pause. Nothing else existed for me outside of what I was experiencing in that moment, and it is still the most intense pain I have ever known.

Without realizing it, my body was moving through the stages of labor much more quickly than I (or anyone else) had anticipated. Suddenly, as I tried to sit still for the anesthesiologist, I pushed my hands against my labor nurse, yelling and moaning from within the deepest part of me.

"I. Can't. Do. This!"

Brendan tried to soothe me. "You can, babe. You can. You're doing it."

The next contraction might have been the worst of all, and I called out from a part of myself that had no plan. "Jesus! Please. I can't." I prayed and cried, but something in me let go too.

I accepted the pain; I surrendered to it.

Though the anesthesiologist was able to administer the epidural, it wouldn't begin working until after our little boy was born. Within a span of thirty-five minutes, I had gone from calmly walking around the hospital with only a few contractions to delivering our sweet baby as he made his way into the world. Sweaty, stunned, and joyous, I held this miracle in my arms and felt deeply proud of myself. My body had experienced intense pain, but I was still standing (well, technically lying—but you know what I mean). Jesus had walked with me; I had not labored alone. But I knew that I'd made the most progress in the moment I surrendered.

This is when pain does its best work.

Surrender is a tricky concept to write about, especially for those of us who have felt powerless over our lives. Maybe a well-meaning friend or family member has even told you, *Why don't you just surrender it?* Although there's some wisdom in that sentiment, there is also potential danger. After all, part of what keeps many of us in a pattern of constantly hustling, becoming overwhelmed, and then finding ways to disconnect is the belief that this pattern is the only way to get through life. We think we *must* control everything. We have experienced environments so threatening that it's laughable when someone presents what feels like a quick fix of "surrender." Wouldn't that just mean giving up?

This is what I mean when I talk about surrender: It's feeling safe enough to release our grip. Surrender can lead us to be gentler with ourselves and others, and sometimes it enables us to ride through the waves of pain that life inevitably brings. When in labor with Jude, the reason I could call on Jesus was because I had begun my journey of trying softer and had come to experience Him as a safe attachment. If I hadn't already connected to Him in that way, I couldn't have convinced myself that God was good in that moment of intense pain. Instead, my cry arose naturally because He had already become my shelter and place of safety.

Paradoxically, when we choose surrender for the right reasons, it empowers us. A curious mystery comes from honoring the truth that surrender with gentleness can be its own form of strength. Our ability to hold our lives with a flexible, open posture allows God's power to manifest in us. As the apostle Paul said, "I will boast all the more gladly of my weaknesses, so that the power of Christ may rest upon me. . . . For when I am weak, then I am strong" (2 Corinthians 12:9-10).

Surrender—when done voluntarily, not from coercion—is a way to be gentle with ourselves, recognizing that trying to control everything can wear us out rather than lift us up. When we give ourselves permission to try softer in this way, our minds can become integrated, our nervous systems are better able to stay within our window of tolerance, and the prefrontal cortex is better able to stay online. We remain attuned to our own experiences, which enables us to connect to our truest selves. From a psychological and physiological standpoint, we are able to move toward integration, wholeness, and peace, open to what may come. Essentially, we grow in our resiliency. The moment I let go of needing to control the pain as my son was being born was precisely the moment when I was able to move through—rather than feel stuck in—the pain.

PART OF OUR HUMANITY

Our desire to try softer, then, doesn't automatically mean life gets easier—it simply means we try differently. Trying softer is not a destination but a way to journey through life. And it's in the trying, in the moving forward—sometimes slowly and haltingly—that we develop resilience. Brokenness and

Try Softer Language

- What is the gentlest thing I could do today?
- What words or affirmations remind me of my true self?
- I wonder if I could take this in smaller steps?
- What would help me stay in my WOT?
- What kind of support do I need to make this happen?
- Whom could I reach out to if I'm feeling overwhelmed?
- How could I help my body feel safe right now?
- What part of myself needs support right now?
- What activity would be soothing for me when I'm feeling triggered?
- Is there a way I could move my body to help me feel more connected to myself?

disappointment are inevitable; resilience is a way to pick ourselves up and fight another day.

I started this chapter as the stomach flu was making the rounds at our house between Christmas and New Year's, that liminal space when no one can quite remember what day it is or what to do with all the big feelings from the holidays. But I embraced that challenging time because I've discovered that internalizing the elements of trying softer often happens not when I'm in the midst of easy days, but in those times when I feel as if I've been pressed down and shaken. And that is why resilience is so critical. Our capacity to be alive grows as we learn to process and move through hard things.

Every sorrow we've grieved, every fear we've felt, every trauma and all the pain we've lived through—it's all valid, and it all matters. More significantly, the hard things that cracked us open have the potential to create space for deeper joy and resilience. As we try softer with ourselves by attending to and listening to our bodies and emotions, we become vast like the Grand Canyon, because our ability to hold the full experience of our humanity increases.

In her famous poem "When Death Comes," Mary Oliver writes of living fully present to the beauty of each person and moment of life. She ends the final stanza this way: "I don't want to end up simply having visited this world."[1]

Oliver's gorgeous words here are like a beacon for all of us who want to do more than survive, who desire the abundant life of which Jesus speaks (see John 10:10). And perhaps this abundance is not made up of wealth and stuff but of awareness, beauty, presence, and connection. Resilience allows us to return to these essentials, even after life has knocked us down.

BACK TO VAGUS, BABY

Throughout the book, we've discussed how learning to practice a gentler way to be in the world enables us to stay in our WOT. But here's the other side of that coin: Once we know how to stay in our windows, we can begin to expand them too. We do this by literally exercising our embodied brains.

To understand how that happens, let's remember how our bodies are designed to handle stress. In chapter 4, we discussed the vagus nerve, the longest cranial nerve in the body that runs from our brains down to major organs like the heart, lungs, intestines, and stomach. You'll remember it is part of the physiology that enables us to stay in our WOT.

In the same way we work to keep other parts of our bodies healthy and in shape, we can actually work to keep the vagus nerve in optimal health, increasing our body's ability to live in our WOT. Dr. Arielle Schwartz describes healthy vagal tone as "an optimal balance of parasympathetic and sympathetic nervous system actions that allows you to respond with resilience to the ups and downs of life."[2] The health of the vagus nerve, then, is essentially a measure of how quickly our bodies can recover to a normal physiological state after experiencing stress. Put another way, the stronger our vagal tone, the easier it is for us to connect with and return to our WOT. Research suggests that healthy vagal tone is related to an upward spiral of mental health and helps us emotionally regulate.[3] When our vagal tone is strong, we can more easily identify when and how we need support from outside ourselves.

So what's the bottom line? Essentially, a healthy vagal tone is the physiological reason behind learning to tolerate (or even enjoy!) experiences that were once overwhelming to our bodies. In a practical sense, this is how our WOT expands. Vagal tone helps us be comfortable with more nuance and recognize that even if something feels intense, it doesn't necessarily equate to something bad. We can learn to rechannel intense energy into fun or play. Gradually, what was once too activating or heavy for us may even become a source of delight.

Mia, another one of my clients, grew up in a chaotic household, and even as an adult, any form of excitement felt triggering. Yet by cultivating her compassionate attention in conjunction with a healthy vagal tone, she has learned to appreciate the exquisite pleasure that comes while attending a sold-out concert or when spending an evening out with a loud but loving group of friends.

In addition to the ways of trying softer we've learned so far, researchers have identified a few other practices that can improve our vagal tone:

- Humming or singing
- Shaking out any part of the body that feels tense or needs additional activation
- Mind/body exercises such as yoga or loving-kindness meditation (see page 206)
- Mind/body therapy (see practices on pages 137–39)
- Diver's response: You can replicate this by splashing cold water on your face while holding your breath. There is strong evidence to show that this practice stimulates the vagus nerve.[4]
- Conscious breathing: See the breath prayer on page 88 as an example.

As we continue the work of trying softer, you will likely begin to recognize situations in which you feel more connected to yourself and others than ever before. You can think of this as a sign that your vagal tone, social engagement system, and WOT are humming along together. In these moments you may even find yourself willing to take risks that feel more like an adventure than a threat.

This was the case for me, and it happened at Disney World, of all places.

BUILDING RESILIENCE

Shortly after Matia was born, Brendan and I had both written off the idea that we could enjoy a vacation before our kids turned five. Parenthood is a lovely gift, but make no mistake, it's the hardest thing we've ever done. Additionally, crowds and intense activity can sometimes be overwhelming for me; over time I've come to realize that because of my past, my nervous system can get revved up even in situations that are *fun*.

When our littlest, Jude, was just four months old, however, we traveled to Florida to see my brother and my sister-in-law and take in a little March sun. They lived about an hour from Disney World.

"We shouldn't go, right?" I said to Brendan. "I mean, I just feel like the crowds would be too much."

"Totally," said Brendan. "It'd be so fun, but no, we shouldn't."

We had both settled into the idea—until three days into our trip, when my brother mentioned Disney World.

"You guys sure you don't want to drive up for the day?" he asked with a twinkle in his eye.

That did it; my adventurous husband was sold, and it wasn't long before I was convinced too. At 6:05 a.m. sharp the next morning, all six of us piled into our rental van and headed to the Magic Kingdom.

With sweet little Jude in my cloth baby wrap—because that's all I'd brought on the trip—we arrived at the park, ready for anything. As we approached the front gate, Tia's eyes lit up with glee. Though Jude slept soundly on my chest, a familiar feeling of overwhelm started to creep over me. *What if? What if?*

When I looked at Brendan, I remembered that we could make this day work in whatever way we wanted. There were no rules as to how to have fun, so we could be as creative as we wanted. And we were.

It certainly wasn't a perfect day. But my thirty-four-year-old self was able to be curious and open to this adventure in a way my twenty-two-year-old self could never have been. Loosening my grip was easier because of all the tools I had learned to use to try softer. In fact, they allowed me to view the intensity of the experience as *fun* rather than *too much*. This was the gift of doing my body-centered work and continuing to grow in my understanding of my body's central nervous and social engagement systems.

Healing past wounds and living out a different story in real time requires new approaches to life. For me at Disney, this meant helping my body negotiate the arousal and seek a visceral sense of safety, even though I was in an intense setting. I don't tell you about my Disney experience because I think the Magic Kingdom will be everyone's key to delight and joy. Instead, I offer it as an encouragement for you to continue in your own work. Where do you see opportunities to reframe something as feeling too hard into an opportunity for fun or adventure?

You may not be quite ready to reframe as "fun" the intense experiences that usually push you out of your WOT. That's okay. But are there ways you can start small? As you become aware of experiencing safety in your body,[5] look for opportunities to build your tolerance of emotion through activities like movement, exercise, or maybe even a good old-fashioned dance party.[6]

Little by little, we build our resilience—until one day, we are doing things we never dreamed possible.

MINING FOR GOLD

You can also grow your resilience by connecting to past experiences that were empowering. This is true even if your story is different than you'd prefer; even if you are still in the process of forgiving yourself for the choices you made to survive. Maybe it's honoring the profound courage it took to live through trauma or survive a difficult family. It might be recognizing that you had the grit to finish your degree. Maybe you acknowledge the resourcefulness you had to find a job, raise kids alone, live with mental health issues, or endure chronic illness.

Think about everything you've survived in your life. These moments are your Ebenezers—"stones of help" that signify what you have walked through and the ways in which God has been with you and loved you every step of the way. And even though you continue to grow and change, dear one, those stones are yours to keep, reminders of how far you've come.

Lately I have been reflecting on my relationship with my mom, which, praise God, is stronger than ever. Recently she came to Colorado for a visit—helping me wrangle my kids, clean our floors, and take care of various other tasks I quite frequently can't keep up with. As I drove her back to the airport for her trip home, she told me, "Aundi, I'm so glad you pay more attention to your kids than to all the details of the house." These days she is *always* looking for ways to repair wounds from our past, finding ways to tell me I am loved right now. And that matters.

She's been sober for more than thirteen years—and it shows. She is anchored, and after years of therapy, AA, and lots of leaning into her own tender story, we can talk about many parts of my childhood that still leave marks. During her visit, I told her that I'd included part of her story—and our journey as mother and daughter—in this book.

"Mom," I asked her, "are you sure you're okay with me sharing what I have in the book? I know it's so complicated, and the last thing I want is for you to hurt more. Honestly, the way you've chosen to own the parts of our lives that have been so hard means a lot to me. I am still healing parts of my own story—but I'm so thankful you have chosen to do your own work."

I glanced at her, and she looked me straight in the eyes. I saw tears as she said, "Aundi, if one tiny part of our story gives someone courage or helps them to know they are not alone in their struggles, then I am more than okay with you sharing.

"I hate that we caused you and your siblings such pain, and I wish I had done so many things differently—but each of you kids is the best thing I've ever done, and I couldn't be more proud of you."

Your story differs from the ones my mom and I tell, but the courage and perseverance you've drawn on just to survive are beautiful too. You can continue to connect with those parts of yourself that are brave and strong. That is the beauty of cowriting a new story with God: We get to choose what to cultivate and what we must learn to forgive in ourselves. I encourage you to see your story through a generous lens. Where are the nuggets of goodness for you to mine? Don't forget these treasures.

So here we are, nearing the end of the book, and we've circled back to where we started: discussing our stories, honoring the full breadth of our lives, and seeing that God can weave together all the pieces.

If you were sitting across from me right now, here is what I would say to you as you continue on your journey:

My dear, you are a shiny, resilient gem who has learned to survive hard things. Now you are invited to thrive.

May you know in the truest part of yourself that you are worthy of giving and receiving love.

May you know that trying softer is your birthright.

TRY SOFTER

Open Hands

You may be familiar with the psalm that says, "Be still, and know that I am God" (46:10). Recently I learned that the phrase "be still" comes from the Hebrew word *raphah*, which means to "slacken" or "to sink or relax."[7] As we consider what it might be like to surrender those things that are either not ours or that are too big for us to carry alone, I want to offer you the word picture of *raphah*, which you can use to soften your posture in proximity to God. It is our invitation to allow the One who calls us *Beloved* to help carry all those parts of life that are too big for us.

If it seems too difficult to surrender yourself to Him in this way, I encourage you to go as slow as you need and simply own and honor this thought: *Just for this moment, I can live with an open posture, knowing God is ever present and gentle with me as I learn.*

"God, Grant Me the Serenity"

Reinhold Niebuhr is the author of the now famous and often recited Serenity Prayer:

> God, grant me the serenity to accept the things I cannot change, the courage to change the things I can, and the wisdom to know the difference.

I invite you to use this prayer as a guidepost in those areas of your life where you may be tempted to white-knuckle it or to take responsibility for things outside your control.

1. In a journal, note those areas of your life where you are pushing harder even though you can't control them. Then take a moment to scan your body and notice if any sensations present themselves. Give yourself permission to simply notice those sensations.

2. If you identify an area you can control, ask yourself, *Is it worth my resources?* We are limited beings, so we must consider where we most want to put our energy.

3. Next, for those areas of your life that you can control and where you are invested, consider how you can ease into trying softer with them so you can stay in your WOT. If you find yourself rigidly sticking to working out or to keeping a schedule or a routine that isn't healthy or helpful, note the ways in which you can gradually try softer rather than white-knuckling it.

4. As you complete the exercise, take a moment to scan your body. What do you notice? Do you feel lighter? Conflicted? Neutral? For now, give yourself permission to simply notice the sensations that come up as you move toward trying softer.

Closing Reflection

Set aside time to reflect on your work throughout this book. I invite you to answer the following questions in a journal:

1. What is your biggest takeaway?

2. What element of trying softer is hardest for you?

3. What practices or perspectives would you like to try to incorporate in your life?

4. What parts of your life can you mine for gold? Consider the times when you have felt connected, empowered, or beloved. Allow yourself to visualize yourself in these moments. What do you notice in your body? What do you see? Hear? Smell? If this experience is comfortable and soothing, give yourself permission to stay in this place.

WE WERE MADE

WITH & *FOR*

COMPASSIONATE

ATTENTION.

BENEDICTION

THIS BOOK, THIS WORK, has been an act of love from start to finish. I hope you feel this truth in my words, for I've lived with too much pain and heartache to skimp on compassion for all of us who are engaged in the process of trying softer.

It is my hope that these words will be a guide, or at least a torch to light your way home. I pray that no matter what, this work taps into the parts of your soul screaming to be loved in extravagant ways. This is simply the truth: We were made *with* and *for* compassionate attention. As you've read this book, I pray your soul has felt a calling, a desire to live the embodied life of the beloved. I pray that as you walk, eat, sleep, cry, laugh, work, and tend to your life, you will sense that in each of these ordinary things you are already deeply known and loved.

I pray that as you do the difficult work of living this life, you will first carry with you the felt sense of your wholeness and your belovedness. I hope you will allow your body—this amazing resource that God lovingly bestowed on you—to inform every part of your psyche, story, and journey. I pray you know that you are in the exact place where God has called you. I hope you will not allow yourself to be satisfied until you have truly tasted and seen the goodness available to you, even if it is only in spurts; even if it feels fleeting. I pray you will hide the hope of it in your heart and use it as a springboard for learning everything God wants to teach you.

I pray that when you get tired in this journey—and you will—you will call on your Jesus and your people. I hope you have the courage to live with vulnerability but also have the chutzpah to set the boundaries you need when a relationship is toxic or hurtful.

I pray you remember to be gentle with yourself as you grow, knowing condemnation never leads us onward but instead stunts the process. May you courageously continue on and move forward in your own story. And when you are weary, may you never—no, never—lose heart. May you know in an experiential, personal, and transformational way that the One who has called you is faithful.

With deep hope,

Aundi Kolber

JANUARY 2019

ACKNOWLEDGMENTS

I'D LIKE TO START BY THANKING my husband and best friend, Brendan Kolber. Without you, it's fair to say this book wouldn't exist—mostly because you've played such a crucial role in my own healing. Brendan, thank you for loving me, holding space for me, and caring for me in this grand adventure. I love you more than words can express.

To Matia and Jude: I want you to know that it is the great honor of my life to be your mom. Writing a book while juggling our lives was not easy, but you helped me remember what matters most. Someday I hope you read this book and know the depth of my love for you. You always have a safe place with me.

To my mom, Maria Kustura: I love you with my whole heart. Thank you for your input as I wrote this book and for your vulnerability in sharing parts of our story. I am deeply grateful for your tenderness and strength.

To my sister, Stephanie Poe: Thank you for being one of the dearest people in my life. I treasure you beyond words, and I couldn't have done this deep work without you. Thank you for believing in me and trailblazing paths of healing in your own right. I am so proud of you, and you and your family are precious to me.

To my brothers—Anthony, Michael, and Jon Kustura—and your families: I love each of you and am thankful for your friendship, love, and support. To my in-laws, Barb and Chris, and all my extended family: Thank you for your continued encouragement.

To my dear friends Lauren Dibenedetto and Sarah Brooks: Thank you for the ways you've loved me in different seasons of this book. To Ashley Abramson: Your friendship has been an unexpected gift in a season when I sorely needed it. To all my friends who've checked in and supported me in this endeavor—I love you.

As they say, writing a book requires a team effort. I'd like to thank my agent, Don Gates, for believing in me. Thank you to my editor and dear friend Jillian Schlossberg; your support allowed *Try Softer* to bloom. Thank you to Kim Miller for your kind and calm guidance. Thank you to Kara Leonino, Eva Winters, Sarah Atkinson, Cassidy Gage, Anisa Baker, Amanda Woods, Jan Long Harris, and the entire Tyndale team for your support and vision.

To my colleagues and mentors and to trailblazers such as Kathy Taussig, John Wilson, Dr. Joannie DeBrito, Mary Ellen Mann, Barb Maiberger, and Dr. Arielle Schwartz: Thank you for your phenomenal work in the therapeutic realm. I am deeply grateful for your influence.

To Michael Cusick, Robert Vore, and Steve Wiens:

Thank you for continually believing in me. To the Redbud writers and the For the Love launch team, thank you for your invaluable support. To my clients and all the folks who consistently show me courage and teach me—thank you.

Finally, to Jesus, who has always been nearer than a breath, who has never left me, and who calls me *Beloved*: Thank you for making a way of healing for each of us.

NOTES

INTRODUCTION

1. At www.psychologytoday.com, you can search for therapists in your area.

CHAPTER 1: "BUT HOW LONG WILL IT TAKE?"

1. While some mental health issues and stressors resolve more quickly than others, for many of us, true healing is measured not in leaps and bounds but in inches. Sometimes this work is done with counselors; other times we do it with mentors, friends, and family.
2. Sarah Bessey, *Out of Sorts: Making Peace with an Evolving Faith* (New York: Howard, 2015), 131.
3. Brené Brown, *The Gifts of Imperfection: Let Go of Who You Think You're Supposed to Be and Embrace Who You Are* (Center City, MN: Hazelden, 2010), ix.
4. This research comes from the Adult Attachment Interview, which essentially measures a person's secure attachment based on how cohesive his or her story is. For more, see Mary Main, Erik Hesse, and Nancy Kaplan, "Predictability of Attachment Behavior and Representational Processes at 1, 6, and 19 Years of Age: The Berkeley Longitudinal Study," ch. 10 in *Attachment from Infancy to Adulthood: The Major Longitudinal Studies*, ed. Klaus E. Grossmann, Karin Grossmann, and Everett Waters (New York: Guilford, 2005), 245–304.

CHAPTER 2: MIND YOUR BRAIN

1. Physiologically, white-knuckling is the antecedent to dissociation. According to polyvagal theory, if fight/flight doesn't resolve a threat, our bodies will resort to dissociation as a way of keeping us safe. This is especially common among survivors of trauma and abuse in childhood.
2. During therapy, I'm not simply observing my clients. When tracking them, I'm allowing myself to use mirror neurons in my brain to experience in

233

my body what they are feeling in theirs. My goal, however, is to remain connected to my (hopefully) more grounded nervous system rather than allowing myself to be swallowed by their experience (e.g., if a client is anxious, I may actually feel tightness in my chest where that person is feeling it). Tracking is significant because children who receive "good enough parenting" from their caregivers experience this and then learn about themselves through the eyes of their caregivers. When children don't receive this, they may grow into adults who are not in touch with their bodies, including the nervous system.

3. For simplicity in this book, I've shortened this response to *fight/flight* or *freeze/dissociation*. However, researchers theorize it can have even more nuanced stages when the sympathetic or parasympathetic nervous system is engaged, such as fight/flight/fawn (Pete Walker). Additionally, according to Schauer and Elbert (2010), the various stages of hyper- and hypoarousal are *freeze, flight, fight, fright, flag,* and *faint.* The first three are hyperarousal, and the last three are dissociation.

4. Pete Walker notes this response comes about as a way to manage and neutralize emotional trauma. See Pete Walker, *Complex PTSD: From Surviving to Thriving* (n.p.: Azure Coyote, 2014), 13. The hyperarousal connected to the fawn response (or what Walker also calls *codependency*) is discussed in Tian Dayton, *Emotional Sobriety: From Relationship Trauma to Resilience and Balance* (Deerfield Beach, FL: Health Communications, 2007).

5. Paul D. MacLean, *The Triune Brain in Evolution: Role in Paleocerebral Functions* (New York: Plenum, 1990), 9.

6. The brain stem connects with your insula in the limbic system to transport information up to your cortex. If the top of your brain is integrated with the brain stem, you can "listen" to what your body is saying. However, if you've learned to suppress or ignore your body, you may still wish to avoid all green rooms, but without any insight as to why.

7. The limbic system includes these structures: the amygdala, hippocampus, pituitary, thalamus, hypothalamus, basal ganglia, and cingulate gyrus.

8. Daniel J. Siegel, *Mindsight: The New Science of Personal Transformation* (New York: Bantam Books, 2010), 19.

9. Siegel, *Mindsight*, 22.

10. Another significant point of integration for the brain is between the right and left hemispheres. For the sake of brevity we're not discussing this here; however, see Daniel J. Siegel, *Pocket Guide to Interpersonal Neurobiology: An Integrative Handbook of the Mind* (New York: W.W. Norton, 2012) for more information.

11. Peter A. Levine with Ann Frederick, *Waking the Tiger: Healing Trauma* (Berkeley, CA: North Atlantic Books, 1997), 45.

12. The reasons we may perceive some things as traumatic include our physiology, past experiences, and how we were parented in and through difficult events.

13. This includes but is not limited to interpersonal, emotional, and shock trauma.

14. I define *metabolize* as the way our bodies process emotions and experiences (including intense or disturbing ones) into moments, ideas, or memories we can reflect on and assimilate into what we've learned.

15. American Psychiatric Association, *Diagnostic and Statistical Manual of Mental Disorders*, 5th ed. (Washington, DC: American Psychiatric Association, 2013), 271.

16. Levine, *Waking the Tiger*, 41–55.

17. Francine Shapiro, *Eye Movement Desensitization and Reprocessing (EMDR) Therapy: Basic Principles, Protocols, and Procedures,* 3rd ed. (New York: Guilford, 2018), 38–51.

18. Stephen Porges, "Stephen Porges: 'Survivors Are Blamed Because They Don't Fight,'" interview by Andrew Anthony, *Guardian*, June 2, 2019, https://www.theguardian.com/society/2019/jun/02/stephen-porges -interview-survivors-are-blamed-polyvagal-theory-fight-flight-psychiatry -ace?fbclid=IwAR31s_VjXwjofKFigWMINCQqxSuLdBVz03q380N6 _BbT_r3l9j9M0V972Ps.

19. Examples I have witnessed in my practice include clients whose caregivers in childhood chronically invalidated their experiences, were hypercritical, or had an active addiction or untreated mental illness. Other traumatic events include growing up in poverty; physical or emotional neglect or verbal or spiritual abuse; loss of a pet; moving; starting a new job; bullying or cyberbullying; racial, ethnic, or sexual discrimination; and medical procedures or crises.

20. Vincent J. Felitti et al., "Relationship of Childhood Abuse and Household Dysfunction to Many of the Leading Causes of Death in Adults: The Adverse Childhood Experiences (ACE) Study," *American Journal of Preventive Medicine* 14, no. 4 (May 1998): 245–58, https://doi.org /10.1016/S0749-3797(98)00017-8.

21. Shapiro, *Eye Movement Desentization and Reprocessing (EMDR) Therapy*, 38–51.

CHAPTER 3: ATTACHED: WHY OUR EARLIEST RELATIONSHIPS MATTER

1. Curt Thompson, *Anatomy of the Soul: Surprising Connections between Neuroscience and Spiritual Practices That Can Transform Your Life and Relationships* (Carol Stream, IL: SaltRiver, 2010), 111.

2. See John Bowlby, *A Secure Base: Parent-Child Attachment and Healthy Human Development* (New York: Basic Books, 1988), 3–4.

3. Daniel J. Siegel, *Mindsight: The New Science of Personal Transformation* (New York: Bantam Books, 2010), 167–89.

4. Ed Tronick, *The Neurobehavioral and Social-Emotional Development of Infants and Children* (New York: W. W. Norton, 2007), 203–4.

5. See presentation by Dr. Allan Schore on YouTube, "Dr. Allan Schore on Resilience and the Balance of Rupture and Repair," PsychAlive, May 13, 2014, https://www.youtube.com/watch?v=cbfuBex-3jE&feature=youtu.be&t=1.

6. For more, see Saul McLeod, "Mary Ainsworth," Simply Psychology, updated 2018, https://www.simplypsychology.org/mary-ainsworth.html. The original source is Mary D. Salter Ainsworth et al., *Patterns of Attachment: A Psychological Study of the Strange Situation* (Hillsdale, NJ: Lawrence Erlbaum Associates, 1978).

7. Daniel J. Siegel, *The Neurobiology of "We": How Relationships, the Mind, and the Brain Interact to Shape Who We Are*, audiobook read by the author (Boulder, CO: Sounds True, 2008).

8. See Kendra Cherry, "The Different Types of Attachment Styles," Verywell mind, updated June 24, 2019, https://www.verywellmind.com/attachment-styles-2795344, which is rooted in Mary Ainsworth's work from *Patterns of Attachment*.

9. Children whose caregivers have been the source of their trauma are put in a tenuous place where they rely on their parents for food, shelter, and care—and yet their nervous systems may be overwhelmed by them. In situations like this, it's common for children with a disorganized attachment style to dissociate.

10. Allan N. Schore, "The Effects of Secure Attachment Relationship on Right Brain Development, Affect Regulation, and Infant Mental Health," *Infant Mental Health Journal* 22 (2001): 7–66; Allan N. Schore, "The Effects of Early Relationship Trauma on Right Brain Development, Affect Regulation, and Infant Mental Health," *Infant Mental Health Journal* 22 (2001): 201–69.

11. Arielle Schwartz and Barb Maiberger, *EMDR Therapy and Somatic Psychology: Interventions to Enhance Embodiment in Trauma Treatment* (New York: W. W. Norton, 2018), 146–47.

12. Siegel, *Mindsight*, 188–89.

13. Because attachment wounds are a type of trauma, certain relational dynamics can "trigger" old wounds. Emotional dysregulation often occurs when our bodies go into fight/flight/fawn or freeze because they are being activated by old wounds.

14. The phrase "good enough mother" was first coined by Donald Winnicott and essentially pointed to the fact that even the most attuned mother wasn't always picking up her baby's cues. However, based on the most current research by Ed Tronick, I now use the phrase "good enough" slightly differently. We know that even the most attentive parents tend to be attuned about one-third of the time; another one-third of the time, these parents are "repairing," or trying to reattune to their children; and the remaining one-third of the time, they are totally out of sync. Therefore, "good enough" refers to the concept that even when at their best, caregivers are only fully tuned in one-third of the time.

CHAPTER 4: TOO HOT, TOO COLD . . . JUST RIGHT: FINDING YOUR WINDOW OF TOLERANCE

1. See Deb Dana, *The Polyvagal Theory in Therapy: Engaging the Rhythm of Regulation* (New York: W. W. Norton, 2018), 104.

2. The *window of tolerance* can also be referred to as the *social engagement system*. I will be using the terms interchangeably in this chapter; however, there is some nuance to each term. *Social engagement system* speaks of the way our bodies are able to interact with other systems—using what is known as the vagal brake—in order to change or affect our state, whereas *window of tolerance* describes the emotional and physiological state we are experiencing.

3. Stephen W. Porges, "The Polyvagal Theory: New Insights into Adaptive Reactions of the Autonomic Nervous System," *Cleveland Clinic Journal of Medicine* 76, suppl. 2 (April 2009): S86–S90, https://doi.org/10.3949/ccjm.76.s2.17.

4. Porges, "Polyvagal Theory."

5. To learn more about polyvagal theory, see Stephen W. Porges and Deb Dana, eds., *Clinical Applications of the Polyvagal Theory: The Emergence of Polyvagal-Informed Therapies* (New York: W. W. Norton, 2018); Dana, *The Polyvagal Theory in Therapy*; Justin Sunseri and Mercedes Corona, *Polyvagal Podcast*, https://radiopublic.com/polyvagal-podcast-WDJmEE.

6. Daniel J. Siegel, *Mindsight: The New Science of Personal Transformation* (New York: Bantam Books, 2010), 62.

7. I picked up this idea from Karen's Twitter feed; she credits Alan Fadling, a spiritual director and author who explores this point in his book *An Unhurried Life: Following Jesus' Rhythms of Work and Rest* (Downers Grove, IL: InterVarsity, 2013).

8. Adapted from an exercise developed by Barb Maiberger and presented during Basic EMDR Training, part 1, by the Maiberger Institute in Greenwood Village, CO, November 2014.

9. Roderik J. S. Gerritsen and Guido P. H. Band, "Breath of Life: The Respiratory Vagal Stimulation Model of Contemplative Activity," *Frontiers in Human Neuroscience* 12 (October 9, 2018): 397, https://doi.org/10.3389/fnhum.2018.00397.

10. Richard Rohr, *The Naked Now: Learning to See as the Mystics See* (New York: Crossroad, 2009), 25–26.

CHAPTER 5: BOUNDARIES BRING US LIFE

1. As Anya discovered, much of what we learn isn't through direct verbal communication. In fact, according to research, only 7 percent of communication is conveyed through words. See Albert Mehrabian, *Nonverbal Communication* (Chicago: Aldine-Atherton, 1972). Many people don't necessarily hear a parent tell them they can't say no. Like Anya, they learn it by feeling shunned, sneered at, or ignored.

2. Henry Cloud and John Townsend, *Boundaries*, updated and expanded ed. (Grand Rapids, MI: Zondervan, 2017), 32–33.

3. Daniel J. Siegel, *Mindsight: The New Science of Personal Transformation* (New York: Bantam Books, 2010), 60. Daniel Siegel points to the idea that mirror neurons only engage successfully when an action seems to have a predictable end (e.g., if someone sneezes, we may start to feel we need to sneeze based on our bodies' mirroring of another person).

4. See Stephen W. Porges, *The Polyvagal Theory: Neurophysiological Foundations of Emotion, Attachment, Communication, Self-Regulation* (New York: W. W. Norton, 2011), 11.

5. Josh M. Cisler and Ernst H. W. Koster, "Mechanisms of Attentional Biases towards Threat in Anxiety Disorders: An Integrative Review," *Clinical Psychology Review* 30, no. 2 (March 2010): 203–216, https://doi.org/10.1016/j.cpr.2009.11.003.

6. Bessel van der Kolk, *The Body Keeps the Score: Brain, Mind, and Body in the Healing of Trauma* (New York: Penguin, 2014).

7. Siegel, *Mindsight*, 28.

8. Joseph R. Bardeen et al., "Emotion Dysregulation and Threat-Related Attention Bias Variability," *Motivation and Emotion* 41, no. 3 (June 2017): 402–09, https://doi.org/10.1007/s11031-017-9604-z.

9. This is referred to as *attentional response bias*. For more information, see Arielle Schwartz, "The Polyvagal Theory and Healing Complex PTSD," August 17, 2018, https://drarielleschwartz.com/the-polyvagal-theory-and -healing-complex-ptsd-dr-arielle-schwartz/#.XRy7TNNKg6g.

10. Adapted from the "I Am Aware" exercise presented by Barb Maiberger during Basic EMDR Training, part 1, by the Maiberger Institute in Greenwood Village, CO, November 2014. During a conversation with Barb, she told me she did not develop the exercise, which is a fairly common mindfulness practice.

11. Body scan adapted from Francine Shapiro, *Eye Movement Desensitization and Reprocessing (EMDR) Therapy: Basic Principles, Protocols, and Procedures*, 3rd ed. (New York: Guilford, 2018), 70, 154.

CHAPTER 6: TRY SOFTER WITH YOUR ATTENTION

1. By some act of grace, I had done a great deal of advanced training around trauma and eye movement desensitization and reprocessing (EMDR) a few years before, so I had a sense that what I was going through could become trauma.

2. Kristin Neff, "The Three Elements of Self-Compassion," Self-Compassion, accessed July 17, 2019, https://self-compassion.org/the-three-elements -of-self-compassion-2/#3elements.

3. Neff, "Three Elements of Self-Compassion."

4. Christopher K. Germer, Ronald D. Siegel, and Paul R. Fulton, eds., *Mindfulness and Psychotherapy*, 2nd ed. (New York: Guilford, 2013), 6.

5. Daniel J. Siegel, *Mind: A Journey to the Heart of Being Human* (New York: W. W. Norton, 2017), 177–79.

6. Nonjudgmental attention has roots in both Christian contemplative and Buddhist thought. For a discussion of the differences between them, see "Similarities and Differences between Secular Mindfulness and Christian Contemplative Practices," Christian Contemplation Curriculum, a joint project of the New Zealand Presbyterian and Anglican Schools' Offices, accessed July 17, 2019, https://sites.google.com/site/contemplation curriculum/home/rationale/similarities-differences-between-secular -mindfulness-and-christian-contemplative-practices.

7. Richard Rohr, *The Naked Now: Learning to See as the Mystics See* (New York: Crossroad, 2009), 59.

8. Daniel J. Siegel, *Mindsight: The New Science of Personal Transformation* (New York: Bantam Books, 2010), 19.

9. "7 Life Lessons from Pema Chödrön," *GuidedMind* (blog), accessed July 17, 2019.

10. Daniel Goleman, *Emotional Intelligence* (New York: Bantam Books, 1995), 13–14, 26, 61–62, 137–38, 144, 203, 211.

11. Andrea Mechelli et al., "Neurolinguistics: Structural Plasticity in the Bilingual Brain," *Nature* 431 (October 13, 2004): 757, https://doi.org/10.1038/431757a.

12. Research also shows that mindfulness increases gray matter in other areas of the brain, including the hippocampus, the posterior cingulate cortex, the temporo-parietal junction, and the cerebellum. For more, see Britta K. Hölzel et al., "Mindfulness Practice Leads to Increases in Regional Brain Gray Matter Density," *Psychiatry Research* 191, no. 1 (January 30, 2011): 36–43, https://doi.org/10.1016/j.pscychresns.2010.08.006.

13. Arielle Schwartz and Barb Maiberger further address why therapists risk burnout and exhaustion if they do not attend to themselves; the same is true for anyone who neglects self-care while trying to attend to the needs of everyone around them. See *EMDR Therapy and Somatic Psychology: Interventions to Enhance Embodiment in Trauma Treatment* (New York: W. W. Norton, 2018), 77–80.

14. John O'Donohue, "John O'Donohue: The Inner Landscape of Beauty," interview by Krista Tippett, *On Being* (podcast), February 28, 2008, https://onbeing.org/programs/john-odonohue-the-inner-landscape-of-beauty-aug2017/.

15. This concept is adapted from the work of Peter A. Levine in his book (with Ann Frederick) *Waking the Tiger: Healing Trauma* (Berkeley, CA: North Atlantic Books, 1997).

16. David G. Benner, *The Gift of Being Yourself: The Sacred Call to Self-Discovery*, exp. ed. (Downers Grove, IL: IVP, 2015), 22.

17. Siegel, *Mindsight*, 61–62.

18. This practice has been adapted from the work of Peter A. Levine in his book *In an Unspoken Voice: How the Body Releases Trauma and Restores Goodness* (Berkeley, CA: North Atlantic Books, 2010).

19. Adapted from Barb Maiberger and Arielle Schwartz, "Somatic EMDR Tools Training," an exercise presented at a training of the Maiberger Institute, Boulder, CO, July 2018.

CHAPTER 7: TRY SOFTER WITH YOUR BODY

1. This idea is inspired by Elisabeth Moltmann-Wendel, *I Am My Body: A Theology of Embodiment* (New York: Continuum, 1994), 1.
2. For more discussion on the intersection of body and spirit, see Tara M. Owens, *Embracing the Body: Finding God in Our Flesh and Bone* (Downers Grove, IL: IVP Books, 2015).
3. Bessel van der Kolk, *The Body Keeps the Score: Brain, Mind, and Body in the Healing of Trauma* (New York: Penguin, 2014), 154–70.
4. Daniel J. Siegel, *Mindsight: The New Science of Personal Transformation* (New York: Bantam Books, 2010), 43.
5. Siegel, *Mindsight*, 44.
6. Siegel, *Mindsight*, 43.
7. Arielle Schwartz and Barb Maiberger, *EMDR Therapy and Somatic Psychology: Interventions to Enhance Embodiment in Trauma Treatment* (New York: W. W. Norton, 2018), 19.
8. This concept originated with Eugene Gendlin in his book *Focusing* (New York: Bantam Books, 1981). I am basing much of my perspective on Peter A. Levine's expansion of it in his book (with Ann Frederick) *Waking the Tiger: Healing Trauma* (Berkeley, CA: North Atlantic Books, 1997), 67–73.
9. Another vital element of the brain that helps us map our own internal experiences and the experiences of others is the anterior cingulate cortex. For brevity, I have omitted discussion of this structure, but you can read more about it in Siegel, *Mindsight*.
10. Siegel, *Mindsight*, 61.
11. Levine, *Waking the Tiger*, 67–73.

CHAPTER 8: TRY SOFTER WITH YOUR EMOTIONS

1. Peter Scazzero, *Emotionally Healthy Spirituality: Unleash a Revolution in Your Life in Christ* (Nashville: Thomas Nelson, 2006), 26.
2. For more discussion on this, see Lisa Feldman Barrett, *How Emotions Are Made: The Secret Life of the Brain* (New York: Mariner Books, 2018).
3. Antonio Damasio, *The Feeling of What Happens: Body and Emotion in the Making of Consciousness* (New York: Harvest Books, 1999), 42, 68, 159.
4. I am referring to a disconnection between our right brains and left brains that can lead to emotional dysregulation.
5. Mitch Abblett, "How Labels Help: Tame Reactive Emotions by Naming Them," Mindful, November 16, 2017, https://www.mindful.org/labels -help-tame-reactive-emotions-naming/; Matthew D. Lieberman et al., "Putting Feelings into Words: Affect Labeling Disrupts Amygdala Activity

in Response to Affective Stimuli," *Psychological Science* 18, no. 5 (May 2007): 421–28, https://doi.org/10.1111/j.1467-9280.2007.01916.x.

6. Daniel J. Siegel, *Mindsight: The New Science of Personal Transformation* (New York: Bantam Books, 2010), 116

7. Siegel, *Mindsight*, 116.

8. Arielle Schwartz and Barb Maiberger, *EMDR Therapy and Somatic Psychology: Interventions to Enhance Embodiment in Trauma Treatment* (New York: W. W. Norton, 2018), 301.

9. If you have experienced significant trauma, it's important that you start small with feeling your sensations; otherwise, you may shoot straight into hyper- or hypoarousal. If this is the case for you, it's especially important to work with a therapist to use resources such as grounding and containment to pace yourself.

10. *EMDR* stands for *eye movement desensitization reprocessing*. It is a mind-body therapy that was developed by Francine Shapiro in 1987 and was originally aimed at only those with post-traumatic stress disorder. However, in recent years EMDR has been found to be a beneficial treatment for anyone who has encountered events or experiences that continue to feel disturbing or traumatic. EMDR uses a specific therapeutic protocol to help neutralize or reintegrate difficult material for various types of issues, including (but not limited to) PTSD, anxiety, depression, chronic illness, attachment issues, transitions, and grief.

11. Barrett, *How Emotions Are Made*, 3.

12. This would be another way to understand what it means to "metabolize" emotion.

13. I was originally introduced to this idea from an exercise presented by Barb Maiberger, Maiberger Institute, Basic EMDR Training, part 1, Greenwood Village, CO, November 2014.

14. When we are disconnected from our emotions, we want to up-regulate, or heighten, arousal in order to bring us into our window of tolerance.

CHAPTER 9: TRY SOFTER WITH YOUR INTERNAL CRITIC

1. Brené Brown, *Daring Greatly: How the Courage to Be Vulnerable Transforms the Way We Live, Love, Parent, and Lead* (New York: Avery, 2012), 71.

2. Dr. Daniel Siegel refers to this as "connect, then redirect," and parenting author Jane Nelsen calls it "connect, then correct."

3. Arielle Schwartz and Barb Maiberger, *EMDR Therapy and Somatic Psychology* (New York: W. W. Norton, 2018), 159.

4. See Kristin Neff, *Self-Compassion: The Proven Power of Being Kind to Yourself* (New York: William Morrow, 2011).

5. Kristin Neff, "Three Elements of Self-Compassion," Self-Compassion, accessed July 25, 2019, https://self-compassion.org/the-three-elements -of-self-compassion-2/.
6. Neff, "Self-Compassion," 47–48.
7. *Strong's Exhaustive Concordance of the Bible*, s.v. "H2617—*checed*," accessed July 25, 2019, https://www.blueletterbible.org/lang/lexicon/lexicon.cfm?t =kjv&strongs=h2617.
8. *Strong's Concordance*, s.v. "H2617—*checed*."
9. W. E. Vine, Merrill F. Unger, and William White Jr., *Vine's Complete Expository Dictionary of Old and New Testament Words* (Nashville: Thomas Nelson, 1996).
10. See 1 Peter 5:6; Matthew 20:16; 2 Corinthians 12:10; and Matthew 5:44.
11. Neff, *Self-Compassion*.

CHAPTER 10: TRY SOFTER WITH RESILIENCE

1. Mary Oliver, "When Death Comes," in *New and Selected Poems*, vol. 1 (Boston: Beacon Press, 1992), 10–11.
2. Dr. Arielle Schwartz, "Vagus Nerve Yoga," December 21, 2017, https:// drarielleschwartz.com/vagus-nerve-yoga-dr-arielle-schwartz /#.XTOGmdNKg6g.
3. See Bethany E. Kok et al., "How Positive Emotions Build Physical Health: Perceived Positive Social Connections Account for the Upward Spiral between Positive Emotions and Vagal Tone, *Psychological Science* 24, no. 7: (2013), https://doi.org/10.1177/0956797612470827.
4. Dr. Arielle Schwartz, "Natural Vagus Nerve Stimulation," July 19, 2015, https://drarielleschwartz.com/natural-vagus-nerve-stimulation-dr-arielle -schwartz/#.XTjGUNNKg6g.
5. If trauma has led to feeling powerless, staying still can feel more unsafe than movement. In this situation, learning to be still in a way that feels safe is also a way to build one's window of tolerance. For more, see Arielle Schwartz, *The Complex PTSD Workbook: A Mind-Body Approach to Regaining Emotional Control and Becoming Whole* (Berkeley, CA: Althea), 2016.
6. If movement has always equated to a threat of safety, high-intensity situations can feel quite triggering. The suggestions offered here are a way to practice "safe mobilization." See also Marlysa B. Sullivan et al., "Yoga Therapy and Polyvagal Theory: The Convergence of Traditional Wisdom and Contemporary Neuroscience for Self-Regulation and Resilience," *Frontiers in Human Neuroscience* 12, no. 67 (February 27, 2018), https:// doi.org/10.3389/fnhum.2018.00067.
7. *Strong's Exhaustive Concordance of the Bible*, s.v. "7503. raphah," accessed August 1, 2019, https://biblehub.com/hebrew/7503.htm.